Choose this not that

for

Gout

by
Personal Remedies

Published by Simple Software Publishing.

Copyright © 2016 by Personal Remedies, LLC
5 Oregon Street
Georgetown, MA 01833 USA

Second Edition

ISBN-13: 978-1490973722   ISBN-10: 1490973729

Printed by CreateSpace.

Choose this not that

for

Gout

Inside this book, you will find a list of food items and easy to follow suggestions on how to improve your health through nutrition and the food choices you make every day.

Suggestions are provided for those with Gout or those who are prone to develop this condition.

In addition, the book contains similar information for those who have one of the following likely health conditions or risks along with Gout:

- Alzheimer's disease
- Cancer risk
- Depression
- Diabetes (Type 2)
- Excess body weight or obesity
- High blood pressure
- High cholesterol
- High Triglycerides
- Stress
- Vitamin D deficiency

Table of Contents

Important Notes

The purpose of this book is to provide helpful and informative material and to educate. It is in no way intended as substitute for medical advice. We recommend in all cases that you contact your personal doctor or health care provider before you embark upon any new diet or treatment of yourself.

This book is sold with the understanding that the publisher, the author and the distributor of this book are neither liable, nor have responsibility to any person or entity with respect to any loss, damage or injury which is incurred as a consequence, directly or indirectly, of the use or application of any of the contents of this book.

How to use this book

The guidelines presented on the following pages are for an adult male or female. They do not apply to children, pregnant women or breast feeding mothers.

Our suggestions are organized by food groups. Within each food group, **items are presented in a specific and deliberate order**. In the case of recommended items (those that could <u>improve</u> your health), the most helpful remedies or suggestions are presented first. In the case of items to avoid (those that could <u>worsen</u> your conditions), the most critical ones to avoid are listed first. The items that are suggested under <u>Instead Choose</u>, are likely to be neutral for your health (i.e., neither improve nor worsen your conditions) based on the information available to us at the time.

Unfortunately, health issues often come our way in groups of two or more. If we are obese or under stress, then chances are we are also at risk with a number of other health issues such as cancer, high blood pressure, or Vitamin D deficiency. If we have Vitamin D deficiency then chances are we either suffer from or have higher risk of getting Osteoporosis, Crohn's disease or kidney problems. Each health issue often results in other health complications, thus the need for looking at a combination of health concerns and risks when formulating our nutrition plans and lifestyle changes. It is for that reason, that we have included separate guidelines for those who might suffer from the most likely and common combinations of health issues related to the main health concern addressed by this book.

One of the factors that make *Choose This not That* series of publications different from all others available to you in the market is that we offer nutrition guidelines for likely COMBINATIONS of illnesses and risks that may be relevant to your situation. We also give you specific guidance by telling you exactly which fish, fruit, vegetable, nut ... is the best for you as well as listing the worst items. We give you an ordered list of food items within each food group, not just a food group.

We have listed alternative therapies and herbal medicines relevant (either helpful or harmful) to your condition. But it is beyond the scope of this book to provide specific guidelines on dosage or how to best benefit from these options. We encourage you to explore these alternatives with your natural health care provider.

Our approach in the *Choose This not That* series is to help people improve or combat their health issues through nutrition (i.e., consumption of food items that they can easily find in their local grocery store), exercise and lifestyle changes. We accomplish that through identification of those items that can improve your health, those that can worsen it, and those that play a neutral role. We trust that you can use this information to alter your diet and lifestyle choices to improve your health and wellbeing.

Serving Sizes

Except for what is noted below, our standard serving size for most foods is 100 grams or 3.5 ounces. For most liquids, it is about half a cup.

For nuts and seeds, the standard serving size is 30 grams (approximately an ounce). For dried fruits, the standard serving size is 25 grams.

For butter, margarine, various oils & fats, fresh herbs (e.g., basil, parsley), crackers, uncooked grains or flour, fresh hot peppers, condiments (e.g., ketchup, mustard, pickles), sugar and salad dressings ... the standard serving size is 20 grams (which in many cases corresponds to one table spoon).

For dry herbs, spices, salt, pepper and the like, the standard serving size is 2 grams (which in most cases corresponds to less than one tea spoon).

Please follow preparation guidelines for herbal supplements, and use a serving size appropriate for the specific use of the herb. Please use caution when selecting these supplements since they are not subject to FDA regulations.

Fruits and vegetables are normally assumed to be served raw. Various fish, seafood and meats are normally assumed to be cooked.

How we developed the content of this book

To provide specific and actionable information and guidance on food choices that you make every day and how they might impact your health, we had to quantify a relative level of goodness (or badness) for every individual food item in our database as they relate to each specific illness or health concern tracked in our system.

Most food and nutrition related research and publications in the U.S. are focused on vitamins, minerals, micro-nutrients, and substances such as cholesterol, fat and fiber. And to a lesser extent there are studies and data on herbal remedies, alternative and complementary medicine, and non-western treatments.

There is not enough data or widely accepted studies that focus on individual foods (e.g., watermelon, white fish and walnuts) and how they relate to specific illnesses or health risks. Our goal has been to help address that void.

Here is a very brief description of our approach:

a) We maintain detailed nutrition information on every individual food item in our system. Most of such data is available from the U.S. Department of Agriculture. And for some data (e.g., Mercury, Gluten) we have found other reliable sources.

b) When there is data available on health benefits (or adverse impact) of a specific food item, or nutrient (e.g., vitamins, minerals) we capture and make use of such data.

c) If a given nutrient is good for a health condition (e.g., Vitamin A is good for night blindness), then all food items that are rich in that nutrient (Vitamin A) are given a positive/higher rating as they relate to that condition (night blindness). Similarly if a given nutrient has adverse impact on a health condition then all food items that contain that nutrient are given a negative/lower rating.

d) Some food items contain much more of a nutrient than others. Our technology takes that into account.

e) Some nutrients are found to be much more effective (e.g., Vitamin A) than some other nutrient (e.g., Zinc) as they relate to a given health condition (e.g., night blindness). Our technology distinguishes between the two.

f) Sometimes a study or a source behind the relationship between a nutrient and a health condition is much more reliable than another. Our approach is sensitive to that.

g) Certain nutrients facilitate absorption of another nutrient (e.g., Vitamin D facilitates absorption of Calcium). We make use of such information. For example, let's say Calcium is good for Tooth Development. Then all food items that are rich in Vitamin D are given a more positive consideration as they relate to Tooth Development.

h) Similarly some substances may reduce absorption of or increase the need for another (e.g., Caffeine may increase the need for Calcium). In the above example, all food items that contain Caffeine will receive a negative/lower rating as they relate to Tooth Development.

i) Our process and the steps mentioned above are automated by our unique (proprietary) and patented technology. At the conclusion of our process, there is a single score that represents the level of goodness or badness for every food item as it relates to each health condition maintained in our system. These scores are the basis for all the sorted lists of food items that you find in the Choose This not That series of publications.

j) For multiple conditions, the sum of these scores is what drives the ranking of the food items and our guidelines.

In closing, it is important to note that in these publications we are not making scientific claims, nor do we suggest perfection of our approach. Our goal is to simply provide a significant improvement over status-quo. No human being or health care specialist can properly and fully take into account the enormity, complexity and contradictions inherent in the interrelationships of food, health, genetics, environment, exercise, lifestyle, etc. that affect our wellbeing. We have merely attempted to use the power of technology to provide you much better and more relevant information to maintain healthier living.

Gout

Gout is a common and painful condition that affects your joints. It is a form of arthritis and can attack any of your joints but it often attacks joints in your big toe first.

Gout is caused by build-up of uric acid in your blood. When uric acid is stored as crystals in your joints, it creates inflammation, pain and stiffness. Uric acid builds up in your blood if you consume too much of certain foods (foods rich in purines), or if your body produces more uric acid than it eliminates. Too much alcohol consumption can adversely affect body's ability to eliminate uric acid in the blood.

You are most likely to get gout if:

- you have a family history of the disease,
- you are a man,
- you are between 40 and 50 years old,
- you drink too much alcohol,
- you are overweight,
- you consume too much of foods rich in purines (e.g., dry beans, certain fish and animal organs),
- you suffer from other medical conditions (e.g., kidney problems, high blood pressure), or
- you take certain medications (e.g., aspirin, diuretics, Niacin).

A Quick Guide to Purine-Rich Foods

Very High (over 140 mg of Purine per 100 grams of food)

- Organ meats: Pork/Beef/Lamb/Veal liver, kidneys, heart, lungs, spleen, tongue; Chicken liver, heart;
- Fish: Sardines; Trout; Tuna; Perch; Anchovy; Herring; Mackerel; Halibut; Salmon; Carp; Pike;
- Seafood: Shrimp; Caviar;
- Beans/Legumes: Black-eyed peas; Soybean seeds; Split peas; Beans (Yellow & White, Pinto, Lima);
- Meat: Lamb (leg); Pork (leg/ham, shoulder, ribs); Veal (loin; shoulder/leg/sirloin);
- Poultry: Goose; Turkey; Pheasants; Quail;
- Other: Liver sausage; Sunflower seeds; canned gravies; Fish/Beef/Chicken stocks & broths;

High (80 to 140 mg of Purine per 100 grams of food)

- Fish: Haddock; Sole & Flounder; White fish; Cod;
- Poultry: Duck; Chicken;
- Meat: Venison; Beef (ground, various steak cuts); rabbit; Pork (cured/ham, bacon); Lamb (ribs)
- Seafood: Scallops; Calamari; Lobster; Mussels; Clams; Oysters;
- Beans/Legumes: Lentils; Chickpeas; Green peas;
- Processed (luncheon) meats: Sausages; Salamis; Frankfurters;
- Grains: Barley; Oats;
- Other: Raisins; Broccoli;

Moderate (40 to 80 mg of Purine per 100 grams of food)

- Peanuts; Cashew nuts;
- Vegetables: Artichoke; Leeks; Brussels sprout; Mushrooms; Spinach; Green bell peppers; Corn; Cauliflower; Kale; Pumpkin;
- Seafood: Eel; Crayfish;
- Fruits: Apricot; Dried figs; Prunes; Banana;
- Grains: Millet; Rye; Whole-wheat;
- Other: Tofu; Sesame seeds; Corned beef; Egg noodles;

Choose these for Gout

Top 5 items to choose:

Cherries & Berries; Water; Juices; Cereals; Yam, Red Cabbage & Peppers;

Food items and actions that could improve your health (within a food group, most helpful items are listed first):

Meat, Fish & Poultry

In general, there is no meat, fish or poultry that can <u>improve</u> your Gout condition. But there are certain food items that may not be as bad for your Gout condition, in particular those fish that are listed at the end of the list of Meat, Fish & Poultry items to avoid.

Eggs, Beans, Nuts and Seeds

Soy milk. In general there are no eggs, beans, nuts and seeds that can <u>improve</u> your Gout condition. But there are certain food items that may be neutral or not as bad for your Gout condition, in particular egg white, nuts and seeds except for the ones that are explicitly listed under food items to avoid.

Fruits & Juices

Cherries (especially tart, including juice); Cranberry juice; Cranberries; Orange juice; Currants; Rhubarb; Cowberries; Oranges; Grapefruit juice; Various Berries; Acerola; Guava; Jujube (fruit); Lemon; Litchi; Longans; Persimmons; Pumelo (Shaddock); Pomegranate; Grapefruit; Kumquats; Litchi (dried); Pineapple juice; Nectarine; Pineapple; Rowal; Natal Plum (Carissa); Currants (dried); Abiyuch; Kiwi fruit; Papaya; Avocado; Peaches; Plum; Breadfruit; Lime; Starfruit; Olives; Pears (dried); Tamarind; Pitanga; Apples (dried); Apples; Apple juice; Tangerines; Mango; Durian; Plantains; Longans (dried); Figs; Peaches (dried); Prunes (dried); Watermelon; Grape juice; Pomegranate juice; Cantaloupe; Honeydew melon; Quince; Figs (dried); Prune juice; Banana; Grapes; Passion fruit; Dates; Pears; Apricots; Apricots (dried); Banana (dried); ***Avoid fruit juices made from concentrate or with added sugar***

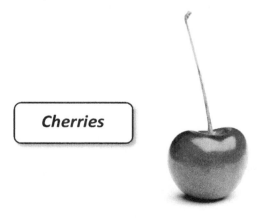

Cherries

Vegetables

Peppers (hot chili, red); Yam; Cabbage (red); Tomato juice; Balsam pear; Balsam pear leafy tips; Garden cress; Lambsquarters; Mustard spinach; Peppers (banana); Peppers (hot chili); Peppers (pimento); Pokeberry shoots; Potatoes w/skin; Sesbania Flower; Taro (Tahitian); Taro leaves; Vine spinach (Basella); Cabbage (green); Amaranth leaves; Squash (Acorn); Watercress; Winged beans leaves; Cabbage (savoy); Borage; Cowpeas leafy tips; Dandelion Greens; Tomatoes; Celery; Bell peppers (red); Kohlrabi; Beet greens; Parsnips; Pumpkin flowers; Squash (Butternut); Sweet potatoes; Swiss chard; Chicory greens; Lotus root; Okra; Purslane; Turnip greens; Onions; Bell peppers (green); Peppers (jalapeno); Arugula; Broccoli; Celtuce; Fiddlehead ferns; Green onions (scallions); Bok choy; Arrowhead; Arrowroot; Artichoke (Jerusalem); Beets; Carrots; Chrysanthemum (Garland); Chrysanthemum Leaves; Cucumber with peel; Endive; Epazote; Fennel (Bulb); Grape leaves; Hearts of palm; Kelp; Lettuce (head); Lettuce (loose leaf); Lettuce (Romaine); Mushrooms (Chanterelle); Nopal; Peppers (ancho); Peppers (pasilla); Shallots; Squash (Hubbard); Squash (Spaghetti); Sweet potatoes leaves; Taro; Tomatoes (sun-dried); Wasabi root; Potato; Brussels sprouts; Broccoli (Chinese); Radishes; Zucchini; Mustard greens; Eggplant; Kale; Garlic; Cloud ear fungus; Mushrooms (Jew's ear); Mushrooms (Morel); Mushrooms (portabella); Mushrooms (shitake); Turnips; Collards; Pumpkin; Rutabaga; Cauliflower; Artichoke; Leeks; Green beans

Breads, Grains, Cereals, Pasta

Various Cereals: rice crisps, shredded wheat, corn flakes, while-wheat, cream of wheat; English muffins (whole-wheat); Bagels; Bread (French/Sourdough); Bread (Italian); English muffins; Tortillas (corn); Spaghetti (whole-wheat); Amaranth; Buckwheat; Quinoa; Toasted bread; Rolls (French); Rolls (Kaiser); Crackers (whole-wheat); Biscuits; Waffles; Rolls (whole-wheat dinner); Bulgur; Triticale; Bread (oat bran); Bread (pumpernickel); Crackers (saltines); Rice (white); Spaghetti; Rice (wild); Spelt; Bread (wheat germ); Bread (cornbread); Bread (white); Oatmeal (cereal); Whole-wheat; Bread (banana); Rolls (hamburger/hot dog); Durum wheat; Rye grain; Bread (whole-wheat); Sorghum grain; Crackers (matzo); Crackers (milk); Crackers (wheat); Pasta; Semolina; Wheat; Bread sticks; Couscous; Melba toast; Wheat bran; Rice (brown); Muffins (wheat bran); Cereal (granola); Oats; Millet;

Dairy Products, Fats & Oils

Fat free or low fat dairy products; Milk (1% fat); Milk (skim); Cheese (Cottage); Whey (sweet); Cream; Yogurt; Buttermilk; Milk (2% fat); Milk (whole); Cheese (Ricotta); Sour cream; Various Cheese; Cheese spread; Cream (whipped);

Desserts, Snacks, Beverages

Water; Popcorn (air popped); Coffee (lowers risk for men, decaf in particular); Coffee (decaf); Pretzels; Potato chips; Popcorn (oil popped); Tortilla chips; Pie crust;

Herbs & Spices, Fast Foods, Prepared Foods

Cornmeal (whole-grain); Tofu; Potato pancakes; French fries; Egg rolls (veg); Macaroni; Parsley; Taco shells; Hash brown potatoes; Corn salad; Croutons; Thyme (fresh); Onion rings; Pizza; Hush puppies; Kimchi; Potato salad; Nachos;

Alternative Therapies & Miscellaneous

Fluids/juices/water; Exercise of various forms including cardiovascular and weight training; Alkaline diet;

Key Nutrients & Herbal Meds

Celery seed; Starch/complex Carbohydrates; Flavonoids; Hawthorn berries; Vitamin C;

Do not choose these for Gout

Top 5 items to avoid:

Fish & Fish Roe; Beer; Brewer's Yeast; Cured & Processed Meats; Fasting; & Excess body weight;

Avoid or consume much less of the following (within a food group, most harmful items are listed first):

Meat, Fish & Poultry (limit daily intake to 5-6 Oz. per day)

Anchovy; Caviar; Fish roe; Herring; Mackerel; Sardines; Scallops; Bacon; Cured meats; Beef jerky sticks; Organ Meats; Beerwurst beer salami; Bologna; Chorizo; Corned beef; Luncheon (processed) meats; Pepperoni; Pork cured/ham; Pork ribs; Salami; Salmon (smoked, Lox); Various Sausage; Beef (ground); Beef chuck/brisket; Chicken skin; Lamb ribs; Goose; Pork; Cisco (smoked); White fish (smoked); Lamb leg; Turkey skins; Pheasant; Quail; Veal loin; Veal shoulder; Beef; Chicken dark meat; Carp; Halibut; Northern pike; Perch; Salmon (pink); Shrimp; Trout; Various Tuna; Walleye; Beef filet mignon; Bison/buffalo meat; Duck (no skin); Rabbit meat; Venison; Lamb; Chicken breast (no skin); Cod; Flatfish (flounder & sole); Haddock; Lobster; Mussels; Squid (Calamari); White fish; Chicken wings; Game Meat; Squab (pigeon); Turkey dark meat; Guinea hen; Turkey breast; Oysters; Frog legs; Eel; Snail; Pompano fish; Sablefish; Clams; Croaker; Crayfish; Abalone; Conch; Various Crab; Cuttlefish; Lobster (spiny); Octopus; Whelk; Various Bass; Bluefish; Burbot; Butterfish; Catfish; Cisco; Cusk; Dolphinfish (Mahi-Mahi); Drum; Grouper; Ling; Lingcod; Mackerel (king); Marlin; Milkfish; Monkfish; Mullet; Orange roughy; Pollock; Pout; Pumpkinseed sunfish; Rockfish; Scup; Seatrout; Shad; Shark; Sheepshead; Smelt; Snapper; Spot; Sturgeon; Sucker; Swordfish; Tilapia; Tilefish; Turbot; Whiting; Wolffish; Yellowtail; Surimi;

Eggs, Beans, Nuts and Seeds

Soybeans (dried); Peas (split); Beans (lima); Lentils; Cashew nuts; Soybeans (green); Alfalfa sprouts; Lupin; Pigeon peas; Beans (pinto); Beans (yellow); Black-eyed peas; Various Beans; Coconut meat (dried); Coconut meat (raw); Chickpeas; Peanuts; Peas (green); Seeds (sunflower); Egg yolk; Pili nuts; Coconut milk; Brazil nuts; Peas (sugar/snap); Egg (duck); Egg (hard-boiled); Egg (raw); Hickory nuts; Macadamia nuts; Seeds: cottonseed, pumpkin/squash, sesame, watermelon, Breadfruit; Butternuts; Chestnuts; Ginkgo nuts;

**Instead choose: Seeds: breadnut tree, chia, flaxseed & safflower; Acorns; Almonds; Beechnuts; Cornnuts; Egg substitute; Egg white; Hazelnuts; Pecans; Pine Nuts; Pistachio nuts; Walnuts;**

Fruits & Juices

Raisins; Sugared Fruit Juice or from Concentrate;

**Instead choose: other fruits & juices;**

Vegetables

Asparagus;

**Instead choose: Spinach or other vegetables;**

Breads, Grains, Cereals, Pasta

Danish pastry; Sweet rolls; Donuts; Muffins (blueberry); Corn; Noodles (egg); Muffins (oat bran); Barley; Croissant; Granola bars; Wheat germ;

Instead _choose_: Corn Muffins; Various Noodles; Oat Bran; Rice Bran; Rice cakes; Spinach Spaghetti;

Dairy Products, Fats & Oils

Milk (chocolate); Hydrogenated vegetable oil; Vegetable shortening; Margarine; Oils: Babassu, coconut, Ucuhuba Butter, Cocoa Butter, Cupu Assu; Fat (beef/lamb/pork); Oils: palm, Shea nut; Poultry Fats; Various Fish Oils; Lard; Cheese (American); Other Oils; Butter; Margarine-like spreads; Non-dairy creamers;

Instead _choose_: Oils: Almonds; apricot kernel, canola, flaxseed, grape seeds, hazelnut, safflower, walnut, wheat germ; Cheese (Limburger);

Desserts, Snacks, Beverages

Beer; Applesauce; Cake (chocolate); Chocolate; Chocolate mousse; Coffee liqueur; Cookies (chocolate chip); Cream puffs/Éclair; Crème de menthe; Hot chocolate; Ice cream (chocolate); Molasses; Peanut butter; Soft (carbonated) drinks; Puff pastry; Carob (candy); Dessert toppings; Red Bull (drink); Candies (peanut bar); Brownies; Ginger ale; After-dinner mints; Cheesecake; Chewing gum; Piña colada; 80+ proof distilled alc. bev.; Fruit punch; Lemonade; Whiskey; Candies; Coffeecake; Halvah (candy); Pie (pumpkin); Eggnog; Pie (coconut cream); Frostings; Jams & Preserves; Jellies; Marshmallows; Pudding; Sherbet; Cookies (butter); Tonic water; Cake (gingerbread); Pie (vanilla cream); Cakes; Pie (fried, fruit); Pie (lemon meringue); Sports drinks; Fruit leather/rolls; Ice cream (vanilla); Cookies; Ice cream cones; Frozen yogurt; Pie (apple); Pie (pecan); Honey; Cake (angel food); Cookies (shortbread); Milk shakes; Pancakes; Taro chips; Malted drinks (nonalcoholic);

Instead _choose_: Potato sticks; Herbal Tea; Wine; Tea; Green Tea;

Herbs & Spices, Fast Foods, Prepared Foods

Foie gras or liver pate; Hot dog; Syrup (chocolate); Teriyaki sauce; Beef broth; Beef stock; Chicken broth; Chicken stock; Barbecue sauce; Tempeh; Tofu (fried); Fish stock; Gravies (canned); Sugar (brown); Sugar (table, powder); Syrups; Miso; Soy sauce; Salad dressings; Chicken Nuggets; Pickle (sweet); Tahini; Soup (beef barley); Soup (chicken noodle); Soup (veg/beef); Ketchup; Soup (clam chowder); Sauce (Hoisin); Cocoa; Sausage (meatless); Falafel; French toast;

Instead _choose_: Cole slaw; Dill weed; Sage; Sauerkraut; Breaded shrimp; Balsamic Vinegar; other Herbs & Spices; Mayonnaise; Mustard; Pickle; various sauces; Vinegar; Cheeseburger; Hamburger;

Alternative Therapies & Miscellaneous

2+ alcoholic drinks/day; Excess body weight; Fasting (for a specific period; don't skip meals); Aspirin; Corn syrup; Deep-fried foods; Smoked Foods (fish); High dosages of Niacin; Prescription drugs (diuretics such as thiazide);

Key Nutrients & Herbal Meds

Brewer's Yeast; Alcohol; Purine; Sugar (fructose); Sugar (refined); Fat (saturated); Molybdenum; Trans fatty acids;

Look-up Table – Food Suitability for Gout

Food Item or Other	Suitability for Gout	Remarks (if any)
1-2 alcoholic drinks/day	Consume less	
2+ alcoholic drinks/day	Avoid	
80+ proof distilled alc. bev.	Consume much less	
Abalone	Consume less	
Abiyuch	More helpful	
Acerola	More helpful	
Acorns	Neutral/OK	
After-dinner mints	Avoid	
Alcohol	Consume much less	
Alfalfa sprouts	Consume much less	
Alkaline diet	Helpful	
Almonds	Neutral/OK	
Amaranth	More helpful	
Amaranth leaves	Most helpful	
Anchovy	Avoid	
Apple juice	More helpful	
Apples	More helpful	
Apples (dried)	More helpful	
Applesauce	Avoid	
Apricots	Helpful	
Apricots (dried)	Neutral/OK	
Arrowhead	More helpful	
Arrowroot	More helpful	
Artichoke	Helpful	
Artichoke (Jerusalem)	More helpful	
Arugula	More helpful	
Asparagus	Consume less	
Aspartame (Equal)	Helpful	
Aspirin	Consume much less	
Avocado	More helpful	
Bacon	Avoid	
Bagels	More helpful	
Balsam pear	Most helpful	
Balsam pear leafy tips	Most helpful	
Balsamic vinegar	Neutral/OK	
Banana	Helpful	
Banana (dried)	Neutral/OK	
Barbecue sauce	Avoid	
Barley	Consume less	
Basil (fresh)	Neutral/OK	
Bass (freshwater)	Consume less	
Bass (seabass)	Consume less	
Bass (striped)	Consume less	
Beans (adzuki)	Consume much less	
Beans (baked)	Consume much less	
Beans (black)	Consume much less	
Beans (fava)	Consume less	
Beans (Great Northern)	Consume much less	

Food Item or Other	Suitability for Gout	Remarks (if any)
Beans (hyacinth)	Consume less	
Beans (kidney)	Consume much less	
Beans (lima)	Consume much less	
Beans (moth beans)	Consume much less	
Beans (mung)	Consume much less	
Beans (navy)	Consume less	
Beans (pinto)	Consume much less	
Beans (winged)	Consume less	
Beans (yardlong)	Consume less	
Beans (yellow)	Consume much less	
Bear meat	Consume much less	
Beaver meat	Consume much less	
Beechnuts	Neutral/OK	
Beef (cured brkfst strips)	Avoid	
Beef (cured dried)	Avoid	
Beef (ground)	Avoid	
Beef brain	Avoid	
Beef broth	Avoid	
Beef chuck/brisket	Avoid	
Beef filet mignon	Consume much less	
Beef heart	Avoid	
Beef jerky sticks	Avoid	
Beef kidneys	Avoid	
Beef liver	Avoid	
Beef rib eye	Avoid	
Beef ribs	Consume much less	
Beef round steak	Consume much less	
Beef shank	Consume much less	
Beef spleen	Consume much less	
Beef stock	Avoid	
Beef tenderloin/Tbone/portrhse	Consume much less	
Beef tongue	Avoid	
Beef top sirloin	Avoid	
Beer	Avoid	
Beerwurst beer salami	Avoid	
Beet greens	More helpful	
Beets	More helpful	
Bell peppers (green)	More helpful	
Bell peppers (red)	More helpful	
Biscuits	More helpful	
Bison/buffalo meat	Consume much less	
Blackberries	Most helpful	
Black-eyed peas	Consume much less	
Blueberries	More helpful	
Bluefish	Consume less	
Boar meat	Consume much less	
Bok choy	More helpful	
Bologna (various)	Avoid	
Borage	More helpful	
Boysenberries	More helpful	

Food Item or Other	Suitability for Gout	Remarks (if any)
Brazil nuts	Consume less	
Bread (banana)	Helpful	
Bread (cornbread)	More helpful	
Bread (French/Sourdough)	More helpful	
Bread (Italian)	More helpful	
Bread (oat bran)	More helpful	
Bread (pumpernickel)	More helpful	
Bread (wheat germ)	More helpful	
Bread (white)	More helpful	
Bread (whole-wheat)	Helpful	
Bread sticks	Helpful	
Breaded shrimp	Neutral/OK	
Breadfruit	More helpful	
Breadfruit seeds	Consume less	
Brewer's Yeast	Avoid	
Broccoli	More helpful	
Broccoli (Chinese)	Helpful	
Brownies	Avoid	
Brussels sprouts	More helpful	
Buckwheat	More helpful	
Bulgur	More helpful	
Burbot	Consume less	
Butter (salted)	Consume less	
Butter (unsalted)	Consume less	
Butterfish	Consume less	
Buttermilk	Helpful	
Butternuts	Consume less	
Cabbage (green)	Most helpful	
Cabbage (red)	Most helpful	
Cabbage (savoy)	More helpful	
Caffeine	Consume less	
Cake (angel food)	Consume less	
Cake (Boston cream pie)	Consume much less	
Cake (chocolate)	Avoid	
Cake (gingerbread)	Consume much less	
Cake (pound)	Consume much less	
Cake (shortcake)	Consume much less	
Cake (sponge)	Consume much less	
Cake (yellow)	Consume much less	
Candies (caramel)	Consume much less	
Candies (hard)	Consume much less	
Candies (peanut bar)	Avoid	
Candies (peanut brittle)	Consume much less	
Candies (sesame crunch)	Consume much less	
Cantaloupe	Helpful	
Capers	Neutral/OK	
Cardamom	Neutral/OK	
Caribou meat	Consume much less	
Carob (candy)	Avoid	
Carp	Consume much less	

Food Item or Other	Suitability for Gout	Remarks (if any)
Carrots	More helpful	
Cashew nuts	Consume much less	
Catfish	Consume less	
Cauliflower	Helpful	
Caviar	Avoid	
Cayenne (red) pepper	Neutral/OK	
Celery	More helpful	
Celery seed	More helpful	
Celtuce	More helpful	
Cereal (bran flakes)	Helpful	
Cereal (corn flakes)	Most helpful	
Cereal (cream of wheat)	More helpful	
Cereal (granola)	Helpful	
Cereal (raisin bran)	More helpful	
Cereal (rice crisps)	Most helpful	
Cereal (shredded wheat)	Most helpful	
Cereal (wheat germ)	Helpful	
Cereal (whole-wheat)	Most helpful	
Cheese (American)	Consume less	
Cheese (Blue)	Helpful	
Cheese (Brie)	Helpful	
Cheese (Camembert)	Helpful	
Cheese (Cheddar)	Helpful	
Cheese (Colby)	Helpful	
Cheese (Cottage)	More helpful	
Cheese (Cream)	Helpful	
Cheese (Edam)	Helpful	
Cheese (Feta)	Helpful	
Cheese (Fontina)	Helpful	
Cheese (Gjetost)	Helpful	
Cheese (Goat)	Helpful	
Cheese (Gouda)	Helpful	
Cheese (Gruyere)	Helpful	
Cheese (Limburger)	Neutral/OK	
Cheese (Mozzarella)	Helpful	
Cheese (Parmesan)	Helpful	
Cheese (Pimento)	Helpful	
Cheese (Port de salut)	Helpful	
Cheese (Ricotta)	Helpful	
Cheese (Romano)	Helpful	
Cheese (Roquefort)	Helpful	
Cheese (Swiss)	Helpful	
Cheese spread	Helpful	
Cheeseburger	Neutral/OK	
Cheesecake	Avoid	
Cherries	Most helpful	especially tart and including juice
Chervil	Neutral/OK	
Chestnuts	Consume less	
Chewing gum	Avoid	
Chicken breast (no skin)	Consume much less	

Food Item or Other	Suitability for Gout	Remarks (if any)
Chicken broth	Avoid	
Chicken dark meat	Avoid	
Chicken giblets	Avoid	
Chicken heart	Avoid	
Chicken liver	Avoid	
Chicken Nuggets	Consume much less	
Chicken skin	Avoid	
Chicken stock	Avoid	
Chicken wings	Consume much less	
Chickpeas	Consume less	
Chicory greens	More helpful	
Chives	Neutral/OK	
Chocolate (dark)	Avoid	
Chocolate (sweet)	Avoid	
Chocolate mousse	Avoid	
Chorizo	Avoid	
Chrysanthemum (Garland)	More helpful	
Chrysanthemum Leaves	More helpful	
Cinnamon	Neutral/OK	
Cisco	Consume less	
Cisco (smoked)	Avoid	
Clams	Consume less	
Cloud ear fungus	Helpful	
Cloves	Neutral/OK	
Cocoa	Consume less	
Coconut meat (dried)	Consume less	
Coconut meat (raw)	Consume less	
Coconut milk	Consume less	
Cod	Consume much less	
Coffee	More helpful	Lowers gout risk for men, decaffeinated in particular
Coffee (decaf)	More helpful	Lowers gout risk for men, decaffeinated in particular
Coffee liqueur	Avoid	
Coffeecake	Consume much less	
Cole slaw	Neutral/OK	
Collards	Helpful	
Conch	Consume less	
Consult your doctor	Most helpful	
Cookies (animal crackers)	Consume less	
Cookies (butter)	Consume much less	
Cookies (chocolate chip)	Avoid	
Cookies (gingersnaps)	Consume less	
Cookies (lady fingers)	Consume less	
Cookies (molasses)	Consume less	
Cookies (oatmeal)	Consume much less	
Cookies (peanut butter)	Consume much less	
Cookies (shortbread)	Consume less	
Cookies (sugar)	Consume less	
Cookies (vanilla wafers)	Consume much less	
Coriander/Cilantro	Neutral/OK	
Corn	Consume less	

Food Item or Other	Suitability for Gout	Remarks (if any)
Corn bran	Neutral/OK	
Corn salad	Helpful	
Corn syrup	Consume much less	Avoid drinks with added sweetener
Corned beef	Avoid	
Cornmeal (whole-grain)	Most helpful	
Cornnuts	Neutral/OK	
Couscous	Helpful	
Cowberries	Most helpful	
Cowpeas leafy tips	More helpful	
Crab (Alaskan King)	Consume less	
Crab (Blue)	Consume less	
Crab (Dungeness)	Consume less	
Crab (snow)	Consume less	
Crackers (matzo)	Helpful	
Crackers (milk)	Helpful	
Crackers (saltines)	More helpful	
Crackers (wheat)	Helpful	
Crackers (whole-wheat)	More helpful	
Cranberries	Most helpful	
Cranberry juice	Most helpful	
Crayfish	Consume less	
Cream	Helpful	
Cream (whipped)	Helpful	
Cream puffs/Éclair	Avoid	
Crème de menthe	Avoid	
Croaker	Consume less	
Croissant	Consume less	
Croutons	Helpful	
Cucumber with peel	More helpful	
Cured meats	Avoid	
Currants (dried)	More helpful	
Currants (raw)	Most helpful	
Cusk	Consume less	
Cuttlefish	Consume less	
Dairy Products	More helpful	Choose low-fat products for gout
Dandelion Greens	More helpful	
Danish pastry	Avoid	
Dates	Helpful	
Dessert toppings	Avoid	
Dill weed	Neutral/OK	
Dolphinfish (Mahi-Mahi)	Consume less	
Donuts	Consume much less	
Drum	Consume less	
Duck (no skin)	Consume much less	
Durian	Helpful	
Durum wheat	Helpful	
Eel	Consume much less	
Egg (duck)	Consume less	
Egg (hard-boiled)	Consume less	
Egg (raw)	Consume less	

Food Item or Other	Suitability for Gout	Remarks (if any)
Egg rolls (veg)	More helpful	
Egg substitute	Neutral/OK	
Egg white	Neutral/OK	
Egg yolk	Consume less	
Eggnog	Consume much less	
Eggplant	Helpful	
Elderberries	Neutral/OK	
Endive	More helpful	
English muffins	More helpful	
English muffins (whole-wheat)	More helpful	
Epazote	More helpful	
Excess body weight	Avoid	avoid low-carb diets
Exercise	More helpful	
Exercise - cardiovascular	More helpful	
Exercise - weight training	More helpful	
Falafel	Consume less	
Fasting (for a specific period)	Avoid	do not skip meals
Fat (beef/lamb/pork)	Consume less	
Fat (chicken)	Consume less	
Fat (duck)	Consume less	
Fat (saturated)	Consume less	
Fat (turkey)	Consume less	
Fat-free or low fat products	Helpful	Dairy products in particular
Fennel (Bulb)	More helpful	
Fennel seeds	Neutral/OK	
Fiddlehead ferns	More helpful	
Figs	Helpful	
Figs (dried)	Helpful	
Fish oil (cod liver)	Consume less	
Fish oil (herring)	Consume less	
Fish oil (menhaden)	Consume less	
Fish oil (salmon)	Consume less	
Fish oil (sardine)	Consume less	
Fish roe	Avoid	
Fish stock	Consume much less	
Flatfish (flounder & sole)	Consume much less	
Flavonoids	Helpful	
Fluids/juices/water	Most helpful	
Foie gras or liver pate	Avoid	
Food prep -- deep-fried	Consume much less	
Food prep -- smoked (fish)	Consume much less	
Frankfurter (beef & pork)	Avoid	
Frankfurter (chicken)	Avoid	
French fries	More helpful	
French toast	Consume less	
Fresh (uncooked) fruits/veg's	Helpful	
Frog legs	Consume much less	
Frostings	Consume much less	
Frozen yogurt	Consume less	
Fruit juice (sugared/concent.)	Consume much less	

Food Item or Other	Suitability for Gout	Remarks (if any)
Fruit leather/rolls	Consume much less	
Fruit punch	Consume much less	
Garden cress	Most helpful	
Garlic	Helpful	
Ginger	Neutral/OK	
Ginger ale	Avoid	
Ginkgo nuts	Consume less	
Goat meat	Consume much less	
Goji berry	Neutral/OK	
Goose	Avoid	
Gooseberries	More helpful	
Granola bars	Consume less	
Grape juice	Helpful	
Grape leaves	More helpful	
Grapefruit	More helpful	
Grapefruit juice	Most helpful	
Grapes	Helpful	
Gravies (canned)	Consume much less	
Green beans	Neutral/OK	
Green onions (scallions)	More helpful	
Grouper	Consume less	
Guarana	Consume less	
Guava	More helpful	
Guinea hen	Consume much less	
Haddock	Consume much less	
Halibut	Consume much less	
Halvah (candy)	Consume much less	
Hamburger	Neutral/OK	
Hash brown potatoes	Helpful	
Hawthorn	Helpful	In berries form
Hazelnuts or Filberts	Neutral/OK	
Hearts of palm	More helpful	
Herring	Avoid	
Hickory nuts	Consume less	
High dosages of Niacin	Consume much less	
Honey	Consume less	
Honeydew melon	Helpful	
Horseradish	Neutral/OK	
Hot chocolate	Avoid	
Hot dog	Avoid	
Hush puppies	Helpful	
Hydrogenated vegetable oil	Consume much less	
Ice cream (chocolate)	Avoid	
Ice cream (vanilla)	Consume much less	
Ice cream cones	Consume less	
Jams & Preserves	Consume much less	
Jellies	Consume much less	
Jujube (fruit)	More helpful	
Kale	Helpful	
Kelp	More helpful	

Food Item or Other	Suitability for Gout	Remarks (if any)
Ketchup	Consume much less	
Kimchi	Helpful	
Kiwi fruit	More helpful	
Kohlrabi	More helpful	
Kola (cola)	Consume less	
Kumquats	More helpful	
Lamb (ground)	Consume much less	
Lamb brain	Avoid	
Lamb heart	Avoid	
Lamb kidneys	Avoid	
Lamb leg	Avoid	
Lamb liver	Avoid	
Lamb loin	Consume much less	
Lamb ribs	Avoid	
Lamb shoulder	Consume much less	
Lamb spleen	Avoid	
Lamb tongue	Avoid	
Lambsquarters	Most helpful	
Lard	Consume less	
Leeks	Helpful	
Lemon	More helpful	
Lemonade	Consume much less	
Lentils	Consume much less	
Lettuce (head)	More helpful	
Lettuce (loose leaf)	More helpful	
Lettuce (Romaine)	More helpful	
Lime	More helpful	
Ling	Consume less	
Lingcod	Consume less	
Litchi	More helpful	
Litchi (dried)	More helpful	
Lobster	Consume much less	
Lobster (spiny)	Consume less	
Loganberry	More helpful	
Longans	More helpful	
Longans (dried)	Helpful	
Lotus root	More helpful	
Luncheon meat (beef)	Avoid	
Luncheon meat (cured beef)	Avoid	
Luncheon meat (pork)	Avoid	
Lupin	Consume much less	
Macadamia nuts	Consume less	
Macaroni	More helpful	
Mace	Neutral/OK	
Mackerel	Avoid	
Mackerel (king)	Consume less	
Malted drinks (nonalcoholic)	Consume less	
Mango	More helpful	
Margarine (salted)	Consume much less	
Margarine (unsalted)	Consume much less	

Food Item or Other	Suitability for Gout	Remarks (if any)
Margarine-like spreads	Consume less	
Marjoram	Neutral/OK	
Marlin	Consume less	
Marshmallows	Consume much less	
Mate	Consume less	
Mayonnaise	Neutral/OK	
Melba toast	Helpful	
Milk (1% fat)	More helpful	
Milk (2% fat)	Helpful	
Milk (chocolate)	Avoid	
Milk (skim)	More helpful	
Milk (whole)	Helpful	
Milk shakes	Consume less	
Milkfish	Consume less	
Millet	Helpful	
Mints	Neutral/OK	
Miso	Consume much less	
Molasses	Avoid	
Molybdenum	Consume less	
Monkfish	Consume less	
Muffins (blueberry)	Consume much less	
Muffins (corn)	Neutral/OK	
Muffins (oat bran)	Consume less	
Muffins (wheat bran)	Helpful	
Mulberries	Most helpful	
Mullet	Consume less	
Mushrooms (Chanterelle)	More helpful	
Mushrooms (Jew's ear)	Helpful	
Mushrooms (Morel)	Helpful	
Mushrooms (portabella)	Helpful	
Mushrooms (shitake)	Helpful	
Mussels	Consume much less	
Mustard	Neutral/OK	
Mustard greens	Helpful	
Mustard seed	Neutral/OK	
Mustard spinach	Most helpful	
Nachos	Helpful	
Natal Plum (Carissa)	More helpful	
Nectarine	More helpful	
Non-dairy creamers	Consume less	
Noodles (Chinese chow Mein)	Neutral/OK	
Noodles (egg)	Consume less	
Noodles (Japanese)	Neutral/OK	
Noodles (rice)	Neutral/OK	
Nopal	More helpful	
Northern pike	Consume much less	
Nutmeg	Neutral/OK	
Oat bran	Neutral/OK	
Oatmeal (cereal)	Helpful	
Oats	Helpful	

Food Item or Other	Suitability for Gout	Remarks (if any)
Octopus	Consume less	
Oil (almonds)	Neutral/OK	
Oil (apricot kernel)	Neutral/OK	
Oil (avocado)	Consume less	
Oil (Babassu)	Consume less	
Oil (canola)	Neutral/OK	
Oil (Cocoa Butter)	Consume less	
Oil (coconut)	Consume less	
Oil (corn)	Consume less	
Oil (cottonseed)	Consume less	
Oil (Cupu Assu)	Consume less	
Oil (flaxseed)	Neutral/OK	
Oil (grape seeds)	Neutral/OK	
Oil (hazelnut)	Neutral/OK	
Oil (mustard)	Consume less	
Oil (oat)	Consume less	
Oil (olive)	Consume less	
Oil (palm)	Consume less	
Oil (peanut)	Consume less	
Oil (poppy seed)	Consume less	
Oil (rice bran)	Consume less	
Oil (safflower)	Neutral/OK	
Oil (sesame)	Consume less	
Oil (Shea nut)	Consume less	
Oil (soybean)	Consume less	
Oil (sunflower)	Consume less	
Oil (tea seed)	Consume less	
Oil (tomato seeds)	Consume less	
Oil (Ucuhuba Butter)	Consume less	
Oil (walnut)	Neutral/OK	
Oil (wheat germ)	Neutral/OK	
Okra	More helpful	
Olives	More helpful	
Onion rings	Helpful	
Onions	More helpful	
Orange juice	Most helpful	
Orange roughy	Consume less	
Oranges	Most helpful	
Oregano	Neutral/OK	
Oysters	Consume much less	
Pancakes	Consume less	
Pancreas	Consume much less	
Papaya	More helpful	
Parsley	More helpful	
Parsnips	More helpful	
Passion fruit	Helpful	
Pasta	Helpful	
Pastrami (cured beef)	Avoid	
Pastrami (turkey)	Avoid	
Peaches	More helpful	

Food Item or Other	Suitability for Gout	Remarks (if any)
Peaches (dried)	Helpful	
Peanut butter	Avoid	
Peanuts	Consume less	
Pears	Helpful	
Pears (dried)	More helpful	
Peas (green)	Consume less	
Peas (split)	Consume much less	
Peas (sugar/snap)	Consume less	
Pecans	Neutral/OK	
Pepper (black)	Neutral/OK	
Peppermint	Neutral/OK	
Pepperoni	Avoid	
Peppers (ancho)	More helpful	
Peppers (banana)	Most helpful	
Peppers (hot chili)	Most helpful	
Peppers (hot chili, red)	Most helpful	
Peppers (jalapeno)	More helpful	
Peppers (pasilla)	More helpful	
Peppers (pimento)	Most helpful	
Perch	Consume much less	
Persimmons	More helpful	
Pheasant	Avoid	
Pheasant breast	Avoid	
Pickle (cucumber)	Neutral/OK	
Pickle (sweet)	Consume much less	
Pickle relish	Neutral/OK	
Pie (apple)	Consume less	
Pie (coconut cream)	Consume much less	
Pie (fried, fruit)	Consume much less	
Pie (lemon meringue)	Consume much less	
Pie (pecan)	Consume less	
Pie (pumpkin)	Consume much less	
Pie (vanilla cream)	Consume much less	
Pie crust	Helpful	
Pigeon peas	Consume much less	
Pili nuts	Consume less	
Piña colada	Avoid	
Pine nuts	Neutral/OK	
Pineapple	More helpful	
Pineapple juice	More helpful	
Pistachio nuts	Neutral/OK	
Pitanga	More helpful	
Pizza	Helpful	
Plantains	Helpful	
Plum	More helpful	
Pokeberry shoots	Most helpful	
Pollock	Consume less	
Pomegranate	More helpful	
Pomegranate juice	Helpful	
Pompano fish	Consume much less	

Food Item or Other	Suitability for Gout	Remarks (if any)
Popcorn (air popped)	Most helpful	
Popcorn (oil popped)	More helpful	
Poppy seed	Neutral/OK	
Pork back ribs	Consume much less	
Pork breakfast strips	Avoid	
Pork cured/ham	Avoid	
Pork headcheese	Consume much less	
Pork heart	Avoid	
Pork kidneys	Avoid	
Pork leg/ham	Avoid	
Pork liver	Avoid	
Pork liver cheese	Avoid	
Pork loin/sirloin	Consume much less	
Pork lungs	Avoid	
Pork ribs	Avoid	
Pork shoulder	Avoid	
Pork skins	Consume much less	
Pork spare ribs	Consume much less	
Pork spleen	Avoid	
Potato	More helpful	
Potato chips	More helpful	
Potato pancakes	More helpful	
Potato salad	Helpful	
Potato sticks	Neutral/OK	
Potatoes w/skin	Most helpful	
Pout	Consume less	
Prescription drugs	Consume much less	diuretics such as thiazide
Pretzels	More helpful	
Prune juice	Helpful	
Prunes (dried)	Helpful	
Pudding	Consume much less	
Puff pastry	Avoid	
Pumelo (Shaddock)	More helpful	
Pumpkin	Helpful	
Pumpkin flowers	More helpful	
Pumpkinseed sunfish	Consume less	
Purine	Consume much less	
Purslane	More helpful	
Quail	Avoid	
Quail breast	Avoid	
Quince	Helpful	
Quinoa	More helpful	
Rabbit meat	Consume much less	
Radishes	Helpful	
Raisins	Consume less	
Raspberries	Most helpful	
Red Bull (drink)	Avoid	
Rhubarb	Most helpful	
Rice (brown)	Helpful	
Rice (white)	More helpful	

Food Item or Other	Suitability for Gout	Remarks (if any)
Rice (wild)	More helpful	
Rice bran	Neutral/OK	
Rice cakes (Brown rice)	Neutral/OK	
Rockfish	Consume less	
Rolls (French)	More helpful	
Rolls (hamburger/hot dog)	Helpful	
Rolls (Kaiser)	More helpful	
Rolls (whole-wheat dinner)	More helpful	
Rosemary (fresh)	Neutral/OK	
Rowal	More helpful	
Rutabaga	Helpful	
Rye grain	Helpful	
Sablefish	Consume much less	
Saffron	Neutral/OK	
Sage	Neutral/OK	
Salad dressing (1000 Island)	Consume much less	
Salad dressing (Blue/Roquefort)	Consume less	
Salad dressing (French)	Consume much less	
Salad dressing (Italian)	Consume much less	
Salami (various)	Avoid	
Salmon (pink)	Consume much less	
Salmon (smoked, Lox)	Avoid	
Salt (table)	Neutral/OK	
Sardines	Avoid	
Sauce (cheese)	Neutral/OK	
Sauce (fish)	Neutral/OK	
Sauce (Hoisin)	Consume less	
Sauce (oyster)	Neutral/OK	
Sauce (pepper or hot)	Neutral/OK	
Sauce (Sofrito)	Neutral/OK	
Sauce (tomato)	Neutral/OK	
Sauerkraut	Neutral/OK	
Sausage (blood)	Avoid	
Sausage (liver)	Avoid	
Sausage (meatless)	Consume less	
Sausage (smoked)	Avoid	
Scallops	Avoid	
Scup	Consume less	
Seatrout	Consume less	
Seeds (breadnut tree)	Neutral/OK	
Seeds (chia)	Neutral/OK	
Seeds (cottonseed)	Consume less	
Seeds (flaxseed)	Neutral/OK	
Seeds (pumpkin/squash)	Consume less	
Seeds (safflower)	Neutral/OK	
Seeds (sesame)	Consume less	
Seeds (sunflower)	Consume less	
Seeds (watermelon)	Consume less	
Semolina	Helpful	
Sesbania Flower	Most helpful	

Food Item or Other	Suitability for Gout	Remarks (if any)
Shad	Consume less	
Shallots	More helpful	
Shark	Consume less	
Sheepshead	Consume less	
Sherbet	Consume much less	
Shrimp	Consume much less	
Smelt	Consume less	
Smoking/Tobacco	Consume less	
Snail	Consume much less	
Snapper	Consume less	
Soft (carbonated) drinks	Avoid	
Sorghum grain	Helpful	
Soup (beef barley)	Consume much less	
Soup (chicken noodle)	Consume much less	
Soup (clam chowder)	Consume less	
Soup (veg/beef)	Consume much less	
Sour cream	Helpful	
Soy milk	Helpful	
Soy sauce	Consume much less	
Soybeans (dried)	Avoid	
Soybeans (green)	Consume much less	
Spaghetti	More helpful	
Spaghetti (spinach)	Neutral/OK	
Spaghetti (whole-wheat)	More helpful	
Spearmint (fresh)	Neutral/OK	
Spelt	More helpful	
Spinach	Neutral/OK	
Sports drinks	Consume much less	
Spot	Consume less	
Squab (pigeon)	Consume much less	
Squash (Acorn)	Most helpful	
Squash (Butternut)	More helpful	
Squash (Hubbard)	More helpful	
Squash (Spaghetti)	More helpful	
Squid (Calamari)	Consume much less	
Starch/complex carbohydrates	More helpful	
Starfruit	More helpful	
Strawberries	More helpful	
Sturgeon	Consume less	
Sucker	Consume less	
Sugar (brown)	Consume much less	
Sugar (fructose)	Consume much less	
Sugar (maple)	Neutral/OK	
Sugar (refined)	Consume much less	
Sugar (table, powder)	Consume much less	
Surimi	Consume less	
Sweet potatoes	More helpful	
Sweet potatoes leaves	More helpful	
Sweet rolls	Consume much less	
Swiss chard	More helpful	

Food Item or Other	Suitability for Gout	Remarks (if any)
Swordfish	Consume less	
Syrup (chocolate)	Avoid	
Syrup (malt)	Consume much less	
Syrup (maple)	Consume much less	
Syrup (sorghum)	Consume much less	
Syrup (table blends)	Consume much less	
Tabasco sauce	Neutral/OK	
Taco shells	Helpful	
Tahini	Consume much less	
Tamarind	More helpful	
Tangerines	More helpful	
Taro	More helpful	
Taro (Tahitian)	Most helpful	
Taro chips	Consume less	
Taro leaves	Most helpful	
Tarragon	Neutral/OK	
Tea (green)	Neutral/OK	
Tea (herbal)	Neutral/OK	
Tea (plain)	Neutral/OK	
Tempeh	Avoid	
Teriyaki sauce	Avoid	
Thyme (fresh)	Helpful	
Tilapia	Consume less	
Tilefish	Consume less	
Toasted bread	More helpful	
Tofu	More helpful	
Tofu (fried)	Avoid	
Tomato juice	Most helpful	
Tomato paste	Neutral/OK	
Tomatoes	More helpful	
Tomatoes (sun-dried)	More helpful	
Tonic water	Consume much less	
Tortilla chips	More helpful	
Tortillas (corn)	More helpful	
Trans fatty acids	Consume less	
Triticale	More helpful	
Trout	Consume much less	
Tuna (blue fin)	Consume much less	
Tuna (canned)	Consume much less	
Tuna (yellowfin)	Consume much less	
Turbot	Consume less	
Turkey breast	Consume much less	
Turkey dark meat	Consume much less	
Turkey giblets	Consume much less	
Turkey heart	Avoid	
Turkey liver	Consume much less	
Turkey skins	Avoid	
Turmeric	Neutral/OK	
Turnip greens	More helpful	
Turnips	Helpful	

Food Item or Other	Suitability for Gout	Remarks (if any)
Veal heart	Avoid	
Veal kidneys	Avoid	
Veal liver	Avoid	
Veal loin	Avoid	
Veal lungs	Avoid	
Veal shank	Consume much less	
Veal shoulder	Avoid	
Veal spleen	Consume much less	
Veal thymus	Consume much less	
Veal tongue	Avoid	
Vegetable shortening	Consume much less	
Venison	Consume much less	
Vine spinach (Basella)	Most helpful	
Vinegar	Neutral/OK	
Vitamin C (Ascorbic acid)	Helpful; May help lower uric acid levels at doses of 500 - 1,500 mg/day	
Waffles	More helpful	
Walk, wheel, or jog	More helpful	
Walleye	Consume much less	
Walnuts	Neutral/OK	
Walnuts (black)	Neutral/OK	
Wasabi root	More helpful	
Water	Most helpful	
Watercress	Most helpful	
Watermelon	Helpful	
Wheat	Helpful	
Wheat bran	Helpful	
Wheat germ	Consume less	
Whelk	Consume less	
Whey (sweet)	More helpful	
Whiskey	Consume much less	
White fish	Consume much less	
White fish (smoked)	Avoid	
Whiting	Consume less	
Whole-wheat	Helpful	
Wine (red)	Neutral/OK	
Wine (white)	Neutral/OK	
Winged beans leaves	Most helpful	
Wolffish	Consume less	
Yam	Most helpful	
Yellowtail	Consume less	
Yogurt	Helpful	
Zucchini	Helpful	

High Cholesterol (& Gout)

Cholesterol is a fat-like substance found in every cell of your body. Your body needs cholesterol to function properly, and it normally produces the amount of cholesterol that it requires. However, many foods that you consume can also result in increase in the level of cholesterol in your body -- in your blood in particular. There is usually no symptom for high cholesterol, but it can be discovered through a routine blood test.

High levels of cholesterol in your blood can result in build-up of what is known as plaque in your arteries. Plaque can narrow or block your arteries. Since arteries carry blood from your heart to the rest of your body, high level of cholesterol can result in heart disease and damage your cardiovascular system.

Cholesterol exists in two forms in your blood known as: LDL and HDL. LDL is called bad cholesterol because it leads to build up of plaque in your arteries. HDL is called good cholesterol because it removes and carries cholesterol away and delivers it to your liver where it gets eliminated from your body.

Your LDL is considered too high if it is greater than 160 milligram per deciliter. Your HDL is considered too low if it is less than 40 mg/dl. Your total cholesterol is considered too high if it is greater than 240 mg/dl, and is considered desirable if it is less than 200 mg/dl.

You are likely to have high cholesterol if you consume too much animal fat and trans fatty acids, you are not physically active, you are overweight, and there is a history of the same in your family. Your cholesterol levels tend to rise as you get older.

Choose these for   Gout & High Cholesterol

Top 5 items to choose:

> Berries & Fruits; Tomato & Cranberry Juice; Cabbage,
> Taro Leaves & other green leafy vegetables; Sweet
> Potatoes & Yam; and Exercise

Food items and actions that could improve your health (within a food group, most helpful items are listed first):

Meat, Fish & Poultry (2+ fish meals per week)

Surimi; Bass (freshwater); Bluefish; Cisco; Drum; Mackerel (king); Marlin; Milkfish; Spot; Sturgeon; Sucker; Swordfish; Tilapia; Tilefish; Whiting; Wolffish; Yellowtail; Bass (striped); Pollock; Snapper; Bass (seabass); Butterfish; Scup; Cusk; Smelt; Mullet; Shark; Sablefish; Catfish; Lingcod; Rockfish; Shad; Seatrout; Grouper; Monkfish; Sheepshead; White fish; Pompano fish; Dolphinfish (Mahi-Mahi); Burbot; Ling; Pumpkinseed sunfish; Turbot; Halibut; Trout; Various Tuna; Flatfish (flounder & sole); Pout; Cod; Northern pike;

Eggs, Beans, Nuts and Seeds

Peas (sugar/snap); Beans: navy, yardlong, fava; Peas (green); Almonds; Walnuts; Seeds (chia); Soy milk; Seeds (sesame); other beans; Chickpeas; Pigeon peas; Lentils; Macadamia nuts; Black-eyed peas; Hazelnuts or Filberts; Peas (split); Seeds (flaxseed); Egg white; Ginkgo nuts; Cornnuts; Seeds (breadnut tree); Pecans; Lupin; Egg substitute; Breadfruit seeds;

Fruits & Juices

Cranberries; Currants (raw); Blackberries; Raspberries; Cranberry juice; Guava; Rhubarb; other Berries; Pomegranate; Cherries (especially tart, including juice); Grapefruit; Plum; Rowal; Kumquats; Tamarind; Peaches; Lemon; Grapefruit juice; Currants (dried); Abiyuch; Watermelon; Avocado; Papaya; Acerola; Jujube (fruit); Litchi; Longans; Persimmons; Pumelo (Shaddock); Nectarine; Mango; Kiwi fruit; Passion fruit; Breadfruit; Lime; Starfruit; Litchi (dried); Pineapple juice; Oranges; Apples (eat with skin); Pineapple; Cantaloupe; Natal Plum (Carissa); Plantains; Durian; Tangerines; Olives; Dried Fruits; Pitanga; Figs; Apricots; Grapes; Orange juice; Grape juice; Pomegranate juice; Banana; Honeydew melon; Quince; Prune juice; Dates; Apple juice (use fresh apples with skin); Pears; Raisins;

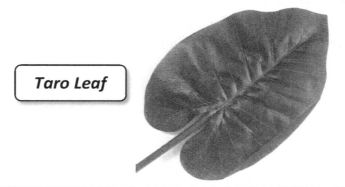

Taro Leaf

Vegetables

Tomato juice; Taro leaves; Cabbage; Peppers (pimento); Dandelion Greens; Garden cress; Pokeberry shoots; Sweet potatoes; Tomatoes; Chicory greens; Watercress; Squash (Butternut); Turnip greens; Yam; Broccoli; Beet greens; Grape leaves; Sweet potatoes leaves; Tomatoes (sun-dried); Balsam pear; Endive; Peppers (banana); Lambsquarters; Mustard spinach; Carrots; Chrysanthemum (Garland); Mushrooms (Chanterelle); Squash (Acorn); Squash (Hubbard); Swiss chard; Winged beans leaves; Peppers (hot chili, red); Peppers (jalapeno); Arugula; Bok choy; Broccoli (Chinese); Kohlrabi; Balsam pear leafy tips; Lettuce: loose leaf, Romaine; Okra; Potatoes w/skin; Sesbania Flower; Taro (Tahitian); Vine spinach (Basella); Green onions (scallions); Parsnips; Mustard greens; Cloud ear fungus; Onions; Amaranth leaves; Peppers (pasilla); Mushrooms (shitake); Brussels sprouts; Lotus root; Borage; Cowpeas leafy tips; Collards; Peppers (hot chili); Kale; Fiddlehead ferns; Pumpkin flowers; Zucchini; Peppers (ancho); Taro; Arrowroot; Chrysanthemum Leaves; Fennel (Bulb); Purslane; Shallots; Mushrooms (portabella); Pumpkin; Celery; Celtuce; Lettuce (head); Nopal; Bell peppers (red); Epazote; Potato; Garlic; Arrowhead; Cucumber with peel; Squash (Spaghetti); Wasabi root; Radishes; Bell peppers (green); Mushrooms (Jew's ear); Kelp; Mushrooms (Morel); Spinach; Artichoke (Jerusalem); Beets; Green beans; Leeks; Turnips; Hearts of palm; Rutabaga; Cauliflower; Eggplant; Artichoke; Asparagus

Breads, Grains, Cereals, Pasta

English muffins (whole-wheat); Spaghetti (whole-wheat); Cereal (shredded wheat); Cereal (corn flakes); Quinoa; Oatmeal (cereal); Triticale; Cereal (whole-wheat); Bulgur; Cereal (raisin bran); Bread (whole-wheat); Amaranth; Buckwheat; Rye grain; Spelt; Whole-wheat; Barley; Durum wheat; Rice (wild); Bread (French/Sourdough); Cereal (bran flakes); Cereal (rice crisps); Sorghum grain; Corn bran; Oat bran (3 grams per day); Tortillas (corn); Toasted bread; English muffins; Bread (oat bran); Bread (Italian); Rice (brown); Bread (wheat germ); Wheat bran; Millet; Bagels; Spaghetti; Oats; Rolls (whole-wheat dinner); Rice cakes (Brown rice); Bread (pumpernickel); Cereal (cream of wheat); Rice bran; Rice (white); Rolls (French); Bread (white); Crackers (whole-wheat); Semolina; Wheat; Corn; Couscous; Cereal (wheat germ);

Dairy Products, Fats & Oils

Yogurt; Oil (olive, extra virgin); Oil (flaxseed); Cheese (Cottage); Milk (1% fat); Whey (sweet); Milk (skim); Cream; Fat-free or Low Fat products;

Desserts, Snacks, Beverages

Popcorn (air popped); Water; Coffee (lowers gout risk among men, decaf in particular); Coffee (decaf); Potato chips; Wine (red); Tea (plain); Tea (green, do not brew or drink tea scolding hot); Popcorn (oil popped); Pretzels;

Herbs & Spices, Prepared & Fast Foods

Cornmeal (whole-grain); Parsley; Ginger; Turmeric; Tofu; Soup (minestrone); Thyme (fresh); Tomato paste; Egg rolls (veg); Cayenne (red) pepper; Cinnamon; Saffron; Coriander/Cilantro; Soup (vegetable); Corn salad; Macaroni; Soup (tomato); French fries; Croutons; Soup (clam chowder); Succotash; Basil (fresh);

Alternative Therapies & Miscellaneous

Exercise; **Fat-free or low fat products**; **Fluids/juices/water**; Glucomannan; Wild fish and free range animals;

Key Nutrients & Herbal Meds

Celery seed; **Psyllium**; Fenugreek seeds; Fiber (soluble fiber); Flavonoids; Omega-3 fatty acids; Starch/complex carbohydrates; Vitamin B-3 (Niacin, for cardio system, in nicotinic acid form, not recommended as supplement or drug); Yucca;

Do not choose these for   Gout & High Cholesterol

Top 5 items to avoid:

Cured and Luncheon Meats; Chocolate; Sweets;
Organ meats; Hydrogenated vegetable oil; &
Excess body weight;

Avoid or consume much less of the following (within a food group, most harmful items are listed first):

Meat, Fish & Poultry

Cured meats; Luncheon (processed) meats; Bacon; Beef jerky sticks; Beef tongue; Chorizo; Corned beef; Pepperoni; Pork breakfast strips; Pork liver cheese; Pork ribs; Pork cured/ham; Beef chuck/brisket; Chicken skin; Chicken heart; Pork lungs; Pork shoulder; Turkey skins; Goose; Lamb brain; Lamb tongue; Pork spleen; Beef (ground); Organ Meats; Lamb ribs; Pork spare ribs; Pork leg/ham; Pork skins; Chicken dark meat; Shrimp; Lamb (ground); Beef ribs; Lamb shoulder; Pork headcheese; Lamb loin; Beef shank; Chicken wings; Quail; Squab (pigeon); Lamb leg; Bison/buffalo meat; Squid (Calamari); Cuttlefish; Venison; Duck (no skin); Pork back ribs; Beef top sirloin; Rabbit meat; Beef tenderloin/Tbone/portrhse; Pork loin/sirloin; Veal shoulder; Lobster; Scallops; Goat meat; Beef rib eye; Quail breast; Turkey dark meat; Turkey breast; Whelk; Beef round steak; Pheasant; Abalone; Frog legs; Guinea hen; Fish roe; Veal shank; Caribou meat; Eel; Veal loin; Beef filet mignon; Sardines; Crayfish; Crab (Blue); Pheasant breast; Crab (Alaskan King); Snail; Clams; Caviar; Octopus; Chicken breast (no skin); Herring; Mackerel; Salmon (smoked, Lox); Lobster (spiny); Oysters; Crab (snow); White fish (smoked); Perch;

Additional options for fish: Mussels; Walleye; Anchovy; Croaker; Pink Salmon; Dungeness Crab; Conch;

Eggs, Beans, Nuts and Seeds

Coconut meat (dried); Egg yolk; Egg (hard-boiled); Egg (raw); Seeds: cottonseed, watermelon, pumpkin/squash; Coconut meat (raw); Coconut milk; Pili nuts; Cashew nuts; Egg (duck); Brazil nuts; Seeds: safflower, sunflower; Butternuts; Soybeans (green); Hickory nuts; Pine nuts;

Instead choose: Acorns; Pistachio nuts; Peanuts; Chestnuts; Black Walnuts; Soybeans (dried); Beechnuts; Alfalfa sprouts;

Breads, Grains, Cereals, Pasta

Danish pastry; Sweet rolls; Donuts; Muffins (blueberry); Muffins (oat bran); Croissant; Granola bars; Cereal (granola); Crackers (wheat); Waffles; Noodles (egg); Crackers (milk); Bread (cornbread); Muffins (wheat bran); Wheat germ; Muffins (corn); Noodles (Chinese chow Mein);

Instead choose: Spaghetti (spinach); Rolls (hamburger/hot dog); Noodles: Japanese, Rice; Pasta; Crackers (matzo); Bread sticks; Crackers (saltines); Biscuits; Melba toast; Bread (Banana);

Dairy Products, Fats & Oils

Milk (chocolate); **Hydrogenated vegetable oil**; **Vegetable shortening**; **Margarine**; **Oils: Babassu, coconut, Ucuhuba Butter, Cocoa Butter**; **Fat (animal, poultry)**; **Lard**; **Cheese (American)**; **Oils: Cupu Assu, palm, cottonseed**; **Cheese (Limburger)**; **Non-dairy creamers**; Margarine-like spreads; Various Cheese; Various Oils; Cheese spread; Cream (whipped); Butter; Sour cream; Fish oil (menhaden); Fish oil (herring); Fish oil (sardine); Buttermilk; Milk (whole);

Instead <u>choose:</u> Oils: canola, safflower, hazelnut, almonds; Fish oil: salmon, cod liver; 2% Milk;

Desserts, Snacks, Beverages

Cake (chocolate); **Chocolate mousse**; **Cookies (chocolate chip)**; **Cream puffs/Éclair**; **Ice cream (chocolate)**; **Puff pastry**; **Carob (candy)**; **Dessert toppings**; **Brownies**; **After-dinner mints**; **Cheesecake**; **Candies (peanut bar)**; **Coffeecake**; **Halvah (candy)**; **Candies**; **Pie (coconut cream)**; **Chocolate (sweet)**; **Cookies (butter)**; **Various Cakes**; **Pie (vanilla cream)**; **Pie (fried, fruit)**; **Frostings**; **Pie (lemon meringue)**; **Chewing gum**; **Peanut butter**; **Fruit leather/rolls**; **Ice cream (vanilla)**; **Cookies**; **Pudding**; **Eggnog**; **Coffee liqueur**; **Crème de menthe**; **Chocolate (dark)**; **Soft (carbonated) drinks**; **Marshmallows**; **Pie (pecan)**; **Pie (apple)**; **Molasses**; **Applesauce**; **Hot chocolate**; **Jams & Preserves**; **Jellies**; **Sherbet**; **Ginger ale**; **Taro chips**; **Fruit punch**; **Lemonade**; **Pie (pumpkin)**; **Frozen yogurt**; **Beer**; Potato sticks; Pancakes; Tonic water; Piña colada; Ice cream cones; Sports drinks; 80+ proof distilled alc. bev.; Whiskey; Honey; Milk shakes; Pie crust; Red Bull (drink); Malted drinks (nonalcoholic);

Instead <u>choose</u>: Herbal Tea; White Wine; Tahini; Tortilla chips;

Herbs & Spices, Prepared & Fast Foods

Foie gras or liver pate; **Hot dog**; **Teriyaki sauce**; **Syrup (chocolate)**; **Soy sauce**; **Salad dressings**; **Chicken Nuggets**; **Sugar (table, powder)**; **Barbecue sauce**; **Syrup (maple)**; **Sugar (brown)**; **Syrup (table blends)**; **Beef broth**; **Beef stock**; **Chicken broth**; **French toast**; **Syrup (sorghum)**; **Cheeseburger**; Breaded shrimp; Chicken stock; Nachos; Pickle (sweet); Hush puppies; Potato salad; Onion rings; Pizza; Hamburger; Sausage (meatless); Soup (chicken noodle); Gravies (canned); Sauce (Hoisin); Soup (beef barley); Miso; Ketchup; Tofu (fried); Cottonseed meal; Sauce (fish); Taco shells; Syrup (malt); Potato pancakes; Mayonnaise; Soup (veg/beef); Tempeh; Fish stock; Natto; Sauce (oyster); Salt (table); Sauce (Sofrito); Hummus; Sauce (cheese); Sauce (pepper or hot); Tabasco sauce; Hash brown potatoes; Poppy seed; Capers;

Instead <u>choose</u>: Cole slaw; Sage; Black Pepper; Dill weed; Rosemary; Corn cakes; Balsamic Vinegar; Various herbs & spices; Horseradish; Pickles; Vinegar; Sauerkraut; Kimchi; Falafel; Mints; Mustard; Pickle relish; Sugar (maple); Tahini; Cocoa; Spearmint (fresh); Sauce (tomato);

Alternative Therapies & Miscellaneous

2+ alcoholic drinks/day; **Excess body weight (avoid low-carb diets)**; **Deep-fried Foods**; **Smoking/Tobacco**; **Corn syrup (avoid drinks with added sweetener)**; **Fasting (don't skip meals)**; Baking using butter; Aspirin; Smoked Fish/Foods; High dosages of Niacin; Prescription drugs (diuretics such as thiazide); Canned foods; Processed or Refined foods;

Key Nutrients & Herbal Meds

Fat, saturated (limit to 7% of daily calories); **Trans fatty acids**; **Brewer's Yeast**; **Cholesterol (limit to 200mg per day)**; **Sugar (refined)**; Alcohol; Omega-6 fatty acid (LA); Purine; Sugar (fructose); Molybdenum; Sodium (salt);

High Blood Pressure (& Gout)

High blood pressure (HBP), also known as Hypertension, is a serious condition and can lead to other health issues such as heart attack, stroke and kidney failure.

Your blood pressure is an indication of how hard your heart has to work to pump blood through your arteries and how much resistance to blood flow exists in your arteries. It is highest when your heart beats, pumping the blood (systolic pressure). And it is the lowest between beats (diastolic pressure).

The blood pressure is often shown in form of a ratio, Systolic/Diastolic pressure, and measured in millimeters of mercury. Your blood pressure is considered normal if the Systolic number is less than 120 and Diastolic number is lower than 80. For example, if your blood pressure numbers are 115/79, you are fine. But if your top number is 140 or higher, or your bottom number is 90 or higher then you have HBP. If your numbers are in between normal and high, then you are likely to end up with HBP unless you take some action to prevent it.

There is no clear cause for HBP among adults. But there are some medical conditions (e.g., kidney problems, sleep apnea), certain medications (e.g., birth control pills) and use of some illegal drugs (e.g., cocaine) that can cause the blood pressure to rise.

You are more likely to develop HBP if you are: an over 55 man, an over 45 woman, black, overweight, physically inactive, under a lot of stress, smoke, drink too much alcohol, eat too much salt/sodium, do not eat enough potassium or Vitamin D, or have a family history of HBP.

Choose these for Gout & High Blood Pressure

Top 5 items to consume:

> **Yam & Green Leafy Vegetables; Popcorn;**
> **Guava, Cherries & Tamarind; Tofu; Peppers;**

Food items and actions that could improve your health (within a food group, most helpful items are listed first):

Meat, Fish & Poultry

Marlin; Swordfish; Snapper; Spot; Catfish; Whelk; Pollock; Sturgeon; Bass (seabass); Snail; Bass (freshwater); Pompano fish; Tilefish; Whiting; White fish; Conch; Seatrout; Bluefish; Sucker; Mullet; Rockfish; Bass (striped); Ling; Smelt; Wolffish; Shad; Surimi; Pumpkinseed sunfish; Burbot; Drum; Salmon (pink); Sheepshead; Grouper; Lingcod; Octopus; Trout; Cusk; Dolphinfish (Mahi-Mahi); Tuna (blue fin); Cisco; Monkfish; Pout;

Eggs, Beans, Nuts and Seeds

Seeds: chia, breadnut tree, flaxseed; Pistachio nuts; Various Beans; Peas (sugar/snap); Seeds (cottonseed); Peas (green); Pigeon peas; Alfalfa sprouts; Seeds (safflower); Lentils; Seeds (watermelon); Soybeans (dried); Black-eyed peas; Chickpeas;

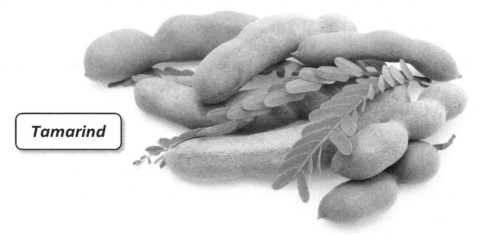

Tamarind

Fruits & Juices

Guava; Tamarind; Cherries (especially tart, including juice); Orange juice; Grapefruit juice; Blueberries; Olives; Plantains; Breadfruit; Jujube (fruit); Longans; Persimmons; Currants (raw); Abiyuch; Durian; Raspberries; Kumquats; Litchi (dried); Lemon; Pomegranate; Rowal; Natal Plum (Carissa); Acerola; Pumelo (Shaddock); Papaya; Avocado; Blackberries; Pineapple juice; Watermelon; Nectarine; Pineapple; Lime; Starfruit; Peaches; Currants (dried); Boysenberries; Cowberries; Prunes (dried); Oranges; other Berries; Grapefruit; Litchi; Apple juice; Plum; Cranberry juice; Pears (dried); Passion fruit; Pitanga; Dried fruits; Prune juice; Cantaloupe; Apples; Raisins; Pomegranate juice; Banana; Tangerines; Honeydew melon; Quince; Kiwi fruit; Rhubarb; Grapes; Mango; Dates; Grape juice; Pears; Apricots; Figs;

Vegetables

Yam; **Balsam pear leafy tips**; **Lambsquarters**; **Mustard spinach**; **Taro (Tahitian)**; **Taro leaves**; **Garden cress**; **Vine spinach (Basella)**; **Amaranth leaves**; **Peppers (hot chili, red)**; **Cowpeas leafy tips**; **Peppers (banana)**; **Borage**; **Winged beans leaves**; **Arrowhead**; **Epazote**; **Grape leaves**; **Various Peppers**; **Tomatoes (sun-dried)**; **Balsam pear**; **Sweet potatoes leaves**; **Arrowroot**; **Squash (Acorn)**; **Purslane**; **Mushrooms (Chanterelle)**; **Cabbage (red)**; **Chrysanthemum (Garland)**; **Chrysanthemum Leaves**; **Shallots**; **Arugula**; **Tomato juice**; **Kohlrabi**; **Cabbage (green)**; **Lotus root**; **Nopal**; **Pokeberry shoots**; **Sesbania Flower**; **Taro**; **Cabbage (savoy)**; **Potatoes w/skin**; **Kelp**; **Bok choy**; **Onions (2-5 oz. of fresh onion daily, or 1 tsp. onion juice 3-4 times a day)**; **Fennel (Bulb)**; **Chicory greens**; **Watercress**; **Mushrooms (Morel)**; **Fiddlehead ferns**; **Green onions (scallions)**; **Bell peppers (red)**; **Broccoli (Chinese)**; **Cucumber with peel**; **Celtuce**; **Pumpkin flowers**; **Cloud ear fungus**; **Carrots**; **Broccoli**; **Artichoke (Jerusalem)**; **Tomatoes**; **Squash (Butternut)**; **Celery**; Turnips; Brussels sprouts; Garlic; Various Lettuce; Wasabi root; Mushrooms (shitake); Sweet potatoes; Radishes; Dandelion Greens; Squash (Hubbard); Beet greens; Mushrooms (portabella); Artichoke; Potato; Mushrooms (Jew's ear); Cauliflower; Bell peppers (green); Hearts of palm; Parsnips; Okra; Zucchini; Rutabaga; Squash (Spaghetti); Turnip greens; Mustard greens; Swiss chard; Eggplant; Kale; Beets; Pumpkin; Endive; Spinach; Collards; Green beans

Breads, Grains, Cereals, Pasta

Quinoa; **English muffins (whole-wheat)**; **Cereal (shredded wheat)**; **Triticale Rice (wild)**; **Cereal (whole-wheat)**; **Spelt**; Bulgur; Bread (whole-wheat); Spaghetti (whole-wheat); Rye grain; Sorghum grain; Millet; Oatmeal (cereal); Buckwheat; Rice bran; Amaranth; Cereal (wheat germ); Oats; Durum wheat; Whole-wheat; Rolls (whole-wheat dinner); Cereal (corn flakes); Cereal (raisin bran); Cereals; Tortillas (corn); Rice (brown); Cereal (rice crisps); Corn bran; Rice cakes (Brown rice); Wheat bran; Rice (white); Spaghetti; English muffins; Corn; Spaghetti (spinach);

Dairy Products, Fats & Oils

Cheese (Cottage); Milk (1% fat); Yogurt; Milk (skim); Buttermilk; Cheese (Gjetost); Fish oil (cod liver); Cheese (Swiss); Cream; Milk (2% fat); Milk (whole); Whey (sweet); Oil (flaxseed); Cheese (Gruyere); Fish oils: salmon, sardine, herring; Cheese (Cheddar); Cheese (Ricotta); Sour cream; Cheese (Port de salut); Fat-Free or Low Fat Products;

Desserts, Snacks, Beverages

Popcorn (air popped); **Water**; Coffee (decaf; reduces gout risk); Wine (red; with dinner); Potato chips; Coffee;

Herbs & Spices, Fast Foods, Prepared Foods

Tofu; **Cornmeal (whole-grain)**; Cottonseed meal; Natto; Cinnamon; Corn salad; Succotash; Fennel seeds; Parsley; Pickle (cucumber); Thyme (fresh); Balsamic vinegar; Vinegar;

Alternative Therapies & Miscellaneous

Exercise; **DASH diet**; **Fat-free or low fat products**; **Fluids/juices/water**; Organically grown foods; Fresh (uncooked) fruits/veg's; Meditation; Pray, practice your religion; Sleep 6-8 hours regularly; Tai Chi; Yoga (certain postures must be avoided);

Key Nutrients & Herbal Meds

Celery seed; **Hawthorn (in berries form)**; Anise seed; Barberry; Calcium; Ginseng (Siberian); Magnesium; Potassium; Starch/complex carbohydrates; Yucca;

<u>Do not</u> choose these for Gout & High Blood Pressure

Top 5 items to avoid:

Excess body weight; Bacon/Cured & Processed Meats; Chocolate; Sweets; 2+ alcoholic drinks/day;

Avoid or consume much less of the following (within a food group, most harmful items are listed first):

Meat, Fish & Poultry

Bacon; Beef (cured brkfst strips); Beef jerky sticks; Beerwurst beer salami; Chorizo; Frankfurters; Luncheon meats; Salami; Pastrami; Sausages; Pepperoni; Pork breakfast strips; Pork liver cheese; Beef (cured dried); Bologna (various); Cured meats; Corned beef; Chicken/Turkey skin; Pork cured/ham; Pork skins; Beef tongue; Pork headcheese; Pork ribs; Lamb ribs; Beef chuck/brisket; Goose; Salmon (smoked, Lox); Lamb tongue; Chicken heart; Pork shoulder; Chicken dark meat; Pancreas; Beef ribs; Organ meats; Pork spare ribs; Liver; Quail; Chicken wings; Pork leg/ham; Pork; Scallops; Lamb; Beef (ground); Tuna (canned); Shrimp; Beef; Bison/buffalo meat; Anchovy; Veal; Duck (no skin); Pheasant; Squab (pigeon); Bear meat; White fish (smoked); Caviar; Fish roe; Quail breast; Turkey dark meat; Sardines; Lobster; Venison; Rabbit meat; Abalone; Guinea hen; Turkey breast; Croaker; Boar meat; Clams; Frog legs; Various Crabs; Squid (Calamari); Goat meat; Beef filet mignon; Cod; Chicken breast (no skin); Haddock; Cisco (smoked); Northern pike; Flatfish (flounder & sole); Crab (Blue); Mussels; Shark; Herring;

Instead <u>choose</u>: *Tilapia; Butterfish; Carp; Cuttlefish; Mackerel (king); Halibut; Crab (Dungeness); Yellowtail; Scup; Sablefish; Walleye; Milkfish; Yellowfin Tuna; Eel; Oysters; Orange roughy; Crayfish; Perch; Turbot; Mackerel; Spiny Lobster;*

Eggs, Beans, Nuts and Seeds

Pili nuts; Coconut meat (dried); Peanuts; Butternuts; Hickory nuts; Beechnuts; Soy milk; Pine nuts; Pecans; Acorns; Egg yolk; Coconut meat (raw); Cashew nuts; Coconut milk; Chestnuts; Macadamia nuts; Cornnuts; Breadfruit seeds; Walnuts; Walnuts (black); Ginkgo nuts; Beans (black); Soybeans (green); Egg (hard-boiled); Egg (raw); Brazil nuts; Egg (duck); Seeds (sunflower); Beans (lima); Beans (navy);

Instead choose: *Seeds (pumpkin/squash); Beans (adzuki); Lupin; Beans (kidney); Almonds; Split Peas; Sesame seeds; Hazelnuts; Egg white; Baked Beans; Egg substitute;*

Fruits & Juices

Avoid sugared fruit juice or made from concentrate.

Vegetables

Asparagus; Leeks;

Breads, Grains, Cereals, Pasta

Danish pastry; **Sweet rolls**; **Donuts**; **Muffins (blueberry)**; **Croissant**; Cereal (granola); Bread sticks; Crackers (wheat); Noodles (Chinese chow Mein); Granola bars; Melba toast; Wheat germ; Noodles (egg); Crackers (milk); Rolls (French); Rolls (Kaiser); Crackers (saltines); Biscuits; Rolls (hamburger/hot dog); Muffins (wheat bran); Crackers (matzo); Muffins (corn); Bread (banana); Wheat; Couscous; Waffles; Noodles (rice);

Instead <u>**choose**</u>: *Bread (French/Sourdough); Crackers (whole-wheat); Bread (oat bran); Bagels; Semolina; Cereal (cream of wheat); Bread (white); Popcorn (oil popped); Barley; Bread (wheat germ); Cereal (bran flakes); Oat bran; Muffins (oat bran); Japanese Noodles; Pasta; Breads: Italian, pumpernickel, cornbread;*

Dairy Products, Fats & Oils

Milk (chocolate); **Hydrogenated vegetable oil**; **Margarine**; **Vegetable shortening**; **Oil (Ucuhuba Butter)**; Non-dairy creamers; Oils: Babassu, coconut, wheat germ, Cocoa Butter, Cupu Assu, palm; Poultry fat; Lard; Oil (cottonseed); Other Oils; Fat (beef/lamb/pork); Margarine-like spreads; Cheese (Brie); Cheese (American); Butter; Cheese (Limburger); Oil (olive); Cream (whipped); Various Cheese; Oil (canola); Cheese spread;

Instead <u>**choose**</u>: *Fish Oil (menhaden); Cheese: Colby, Gouda, Mozzarella;*

Desserts, Snacks, Beverages

Cake (chocolate); **Chocolate (sweet)**; **Chocolate mousse**; **Coffee liqueur**; **Cookies (chocolate chip)**; **Cream puffs/Éclair**; **Ice cream (chocolate)**; **Peanut butter**; **Puff pastry**; **Brownies**; **Dessert toppings**; **Cheesecake**; **Hot chocolate**; **Candies (peanut brittle)**; **Coffeecake**; **Red Bull (drink)**; **Crème de menthe**; **Cookies**; **Pie (vanilla cream)**; **Cakes**; **Pie (coconut cream)**; **Various Pies**; **After-dinner mints**; **Pudding**; **Frostings**; **Candies (peanut bar)**; **Ice cream cones**; **Soft (carbonated) drinks**; **Applesauce**; **Chewing gum**; **Candies**; **Fruit punch**; **Ginger ale**; **Piña colada**; **Fruit leather/rolls**; **Beer**; **Carob (candy)**; **80+ proof distilled alc. bev.**; **Lemonade**; **Jams & Preserves**; **Sherbet**; **Halvah (candy)**; **Ice cream (vanilla)**; Candies (hard); Marshmallows; Eggnog; Whiskey; Jellies; Pancakes; Tonic water; Pie crust; Chocolate (dark); Sports drinks; Frozen yogurt; Potato sticks; Taro chips; Tea (plain); Honey; Milk shakes; Malted drinks (nonalcoholic); Tea (green); Pretzels;

Instead <u>**choose**</u>: *Tortilla chips; Popcorn (oil popped); Molasses; Tea (herbal); Candies (sesame crunch); Wine (white);*

Herbs & Spices, Fast Foods, Prepared Foods

Foie gras or liver pate; **Teriyaki sauce**; **Syrup (chocolate)**; **Hot dog**; **Soy sauce**; **Salad dressings**; **Chicken Nuggets**; **Barbecue sauce**; **Sugar (table, powder)**; **Miso**; **Sugar (brown)**; **Syrup (table blends)**; **Sausage (meatless)**; **Soup (beef barley)**; **Tahini**; Salt (table); Beef & Chicken Broth/Stocks; Breaded shrimp; Onion rings; Potato salad; Sauce (Hoisin); Syrup (maple); Pizza; Gravies (canned); Syrup (malt); Pickle (sweet); Sauce (fish); Ketchup; Tofu (fried); Nachos; Soup (chicken noodle); Soup (veg/beef); French toast; Fish stock; Cheeseburger; Soup (clam chowder); Hamburger; Sauce (oyster); Mayonnaise; Hush puppies; Sauce (Sofrito); Hash brown potatoes; Soup (vegetable); Hummus; Poppy seed; Capers; Tempeh; Turmeric; Sauce (pepper or hot); Tabasco sauce; Croutons; Sauce (cheese); Cole slaw; Mustard; Cloves;

Instead <u>*choose*</u>*: Cocoa; Mints; Potato pancakes; Tomato paste; Pickle relish; Sauerkraut; Falafel; Dill weed; Sage; Soup (minestrone); Corn cakes; Egg rolls (veg); various herbs & spices; Horseradish; Sugar (maple); Taco shells; Tomato soup & sauce; Macaroni; Kimchi; Sorghum syrup; French fries;*

Alternative Therapies & Miscellaneous

2+ alcoholic drinks/day; **Excess body weight**; **Prescription drugs (diuretics such as thiazide)**; **Corn syrup**; **Fasting (i.e., do not skip meals)**; Smoking/Tobacco; Deep fried foods; Aspirin; Smoked Fish/Foods; High dosages of Niacin; Hyperthermia (avoid if extremely high blood pressure); Stress;

Key Nutrients & Herbal Meds

Alcohol; **Brewer's Yeast**; **Sugar (refined)**; Caffeine; Fat (saturated); Licorice; Purine; Sodium (salt; use spices instead or unrefined real salt/sea salt); Sugar (fructose);

High Triglycerides (& Gout)

Triglycerides are a type of fat that exist in the bloodstream, in fat tissues and in foods. Triglycerides can be produced from fats in the foods we consume, from carbohydrates, or from calories not used by the tissues immediately after consumption and stored in the fat cells for future use.

High level of triglycerides in the blood can result in hardening and narrowing of arteries, leading to greater possibility of heart attack and strokes. This condition often occurs along with high level of cholesterol in the blood stream. It is often discovered in the same blood test that measures cholesterol level. Triglycerides level is considered high if it is greater than 200 milligrams per deci-liter.

The most likely causes for having high triglycerides are:

- drinking too much alcohol,
- being overweight,
- consuming too much sugars and carbohydrates
- suffering from other medical conditions such as diabetes or kidney failure

Proper nutrition and exercise can be very effective in lowering the triglycerides level in your blood.

Choose these for Gout & High Triglycerides

Top 5 items to choose:

Exercise; Fluids, Water & Juices; Peppers & Green Leafy Vegetables; Garlic & Onions; Fish Oil; Cranberries & Rhubarb;

Food items and actions that could improve your health (within a food group, most helpful items are listed first):

Meat, Fish & Poultry

Bluefish; Mackerel (king); Marlin; Spot; Sturgeon; Swordfish; Tilefish; Sablefish; Bass (striped); Smelt; Bass (seabass); Wolffish; Pollock; Sucker; Mullet; Bass (freshwater); Drum; White fish; Whiting; Surimi; Shad; Lobster (spiny); Milkfish; Yellowtail; Cisco; Crab (Dungeness); Salmon (pink); Trout; Tuna (blue fin); Mussels; Crab (Alaskan King); Oysters; Tilapia; Crab (snow); Dolphinfish (Mahi-Mahi); Seatrout;

Eggs, Beans, Nuts and Seeds

Seeds (chia); Egg substitute;

Fruits & Juices

Cranberries; Orange juice; Cranberry juice; Rhubarb; Cherries (especially tart, including juice); Currants (raw); Cowberries; Blackberries; Raspberries; Oranges; Grapefruit juice; Other Berries; Acerola; Lemon; Pumelo (Shaddock); Guava; Jujube (fruit); Natal Plum (Carissa); Grapefruit; Persimmons; Pineapple juice; Nectarine; Pineapple; Lime; Starfruit; Olives; Kumquats; Pomegranate; Kiwi fruit; Papaya; Pitanga; Peaches; Plum; Litchi; Abiyuch; Rowal; Apple juice; Litchi (dried); Longans; Durian; Apples; Breadfruit; Tangerines; Currants (dried); Mango; Watermelon; Apples (dried); Pears (dried); Grape juice; Pomegranate juice; Prunes (dried); Cantaloupe; Honeydew melon; **_Avoid fruit juices made from concentrate or sugared_**

Vegetables

Peppers (hot chili, red); Winged beans leaves; Peppers (pimento); Garlic; Taro leaves; Onions; Peppers (hot chili); Cabbage (red); Yam; Tomato juice; Balsam pear; Balsam pear leafy tips; Garden cress; Lambsquarters; Mustard spinach; Peppers (banana); Pokeberry shoots; Sesbania Flower; Taro (Tahitian); Vine spinach (Basella); Squash (Acorn); Mushrooms (Chanterelle); Cabbage (green); Amaranth leaves; Watercress; Potatoes w/skin; Cabbage (savoy); Chicory greens; Borage; Cowpeas leafy tips; Dandelion Greens; Tomatoes; Peppers (jalapeno); Celery; Bell peppers (red); Kohlrabi; Beet greens; Pumpkin flowers; Squash (Butternut); Swiss chard; Fiddlehead ferns; Parsnips; Mushrooms (shitake); Okra; Purslane; Arrowroot; Broccoli; Turnip greens; Tomatoes (sun-dried); Mushrooms (portabella); Sweet potatoes; Bell peppers (green); Endive; Kelp; Arugula; Celtuce; Green onions (scallions); Lotus root; Bok choy; Carrots; Chrysanthemum (Garland); Chrysanthemum Leaves; Cucumber with peel; Epazote; Fennel (Bulb); Hearts of palm; Various Lettuce; Nopal; Peppers (pasilla); Squash (Hubbard); Squash (Spaghetti); Sweet potatoes leaves; Wasabi root; Grape leaves; Artichoke; Brussels sprouts; Potato; Arrowhead; Beets; Taro; Broccoli (Chinese); Mushrooms (Jew's ear); Radishes; Zucchini; Cloud ear fungus; Mushrooms (Morel); Mustard greens; Eggplant; Artichoke (Jerusalem); Shallots; Kale; Turnips; Collards; Pumpkin; Rutabaga;

Breads, Grains, Cereals, Pasta

Cereal (rice crisps); Cereal (corn flakes); Bread (French/Sourdough); Cereal (shredded wheat); Cereal (cream of wheat); Buckwheat; English muffins (whole-wheat); Cereal (whole-wheat); Triticale; Rice (white); Spaghetti (whole-wheat); Toasted bread; Whole-wheat; Bread (wheat germ); Bagels; English muffins; Amaranth; Quinoa; Bread (Italian); Durum wheat; Rolls (French); Spaghetti; Wheat bran; Bulgur; Rice (wild); Rye grain; Tortillas (corn); Spelt; Sorghum grain; Bread (oat bran); Semolina; Oats; Oatmeal (cereal); Rice bran; Crackers (matzo); Wheat; Rice cakes (Brown rice);

Dairy Products, Fats & Oils

Fish oil (salmon); Fish oil (various); Cheese (Cottage); Oil (olive); Oil (flaxseed); Cream; Yogurt; Milk (1% fat); Whey (sweet); Low-fat products;

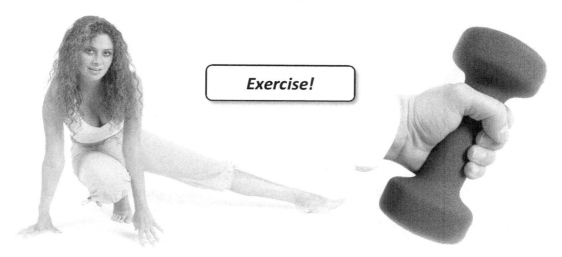

Exercise!

Desserts, Snacks, Beverages

Water; Coffee (lowers Gout risk for men, decaf in particular); Coffee (decaf); Pretzels; Tea (green);

Herbs & Spices, Fast Foods, Prepared Foods

Ginger; Parsley; Cornmeal (whole-grain); Tofu; Cayenne (red) pepper; Cinnamon; Macaroni; Corn salad; Kimchi; Croutons; Thyme (fresh);

Alternative Therapies & Miscellaneous

Exercise (i.e., cardiovascular, weight training, walking, cycling, or jogging); Wild fish and free range animals;

Key Nutrients & Herbal Meds

Omega-3 fatty acids; Celery seed; Starch/complex carbohydrates; Vitamin B-3 (Niacin in Nicotinic acid form);

Do not choose these for Gout & High Triglycerides

Top 5 items to avoid:

Chocolate; Luncheon (processed) meats; Organ meats; Molasses; Sweets/Syrups; Excess body weight;

Avoid or consume much less of the following (within a food group, most harmful items are listed first):

Meat, Fish & Poultry

Bacon; Beef (cured brkfst strips); Beef jerky sticks; Beef kidneys; Beef tongue; Beerwurst beer salami; Bologna (various); Chorizo; Frankfurters; Luncheon meats; Pepperoni; Pork breakfast strips; Pork ribs; Salami; Sausages; Chicken skin; Pork liver cheese; Pastrami (turkey); Organ meats; Goose; Turkey skins; Lamb ribs; Beef chuck/brisket; Pork shoulder; Pork spare ribs; Beef (ground); Pork skins; Corned beef; Pastrami (cured beef); Pork leg/ham; Beef (cured dried); Pork; Beef ribs; Chicken wings; Chicken dark meat; Lamb; Quail; Beef shank; Squab (pigeon); Game meat; Bison/buffalo meat; Sardines; Beef; Pheasant; Duck (no skin); Croaker; Rabbit meat; Veal shoulder; Boar meat; Scallops; Goat meat; Frog legs; Venison; Fish roe; Guinea hen; Turkey dark meat; Tuna (canned); Shrimp; Beef filet mignon; Veal; Squid (Calamari); Turkey breast; White fish (smoked); Eel; Northern pike; Abalone; Perch; Carp; Whelk; Cod; Haddock; Snail; Shark; Crayfish; Veal shank; Walleye; Lobster; Chicken breast (no skin); Cuttlefish; Flatfish (flounder & sole); Conch; Crab (Blue); Orange roughy; Pout; Turbot; Pumpkinseed sunfish;

Instead **choose**: Pompano fish; Grouper; Snapper; Clams; Cisco (smoked); Butterfish; Scup; Tuna (yellowfin); Halibut; Octopus; Catfish; Lingcod; Burbot; Rockfish; Cusk; Anchovy; Mackerel; Herring; Caviar; Ling; Monkfish; Salmon (smoked, lox); Sheepshead;

Eggs, Beans, Nuts and Seeds

Cashew nuts; Egg yolk; Pili nuts; Brazil nuts; Coconut meat (dried); Peanuts; Seeds (sunflower); Hickory nuts; Seeds: cottonseed, pumpkin/squash, sesame, watermelon; Butternuts; Coconut meat (raw); Pine nuts; Seeds (safflower); Almonds; Beechnuts; Pecans; Pistachio nuts; Egg (hard-boiled); Walnuts (black); Egg (raw); Chickpeas; Walnuts; Hazelnuts or Filberts; Soybeans (green); Beans (baked); Lupin; Acorns; Egg (duck); Peas (split); Beans (winged); Coconut milk; Beans (lima); Pigeon peas; Lentils; other Beans; Black-eyed peas; Alfalfa sprouts; Cornnuts; Chestnuts; Peas (green); Macadamia nuts;

Instead **choose**: Seeds: Flaxseed, breadnut; Egg white; Peas (sugar/snap); Ginkgo nuts; Soybeans (dried); Breadfruit seeds;

Fruits & Juices

Raisins; Dates; Apricots (dried); Banana (dried); Avoid fruit Juice from concentrate or sugared;

Instead **choose**: Longans (dried); Peaches (dried); Plantains; Figs; Quince; Passion fruit; Avocado; Apricots; Figs (dried); Banana; Tamarind; Pears; Prune juice; Elderberries; Grapes;

Vegetables

Asparagus;

Instead choose: Leeks; Green beans; Spinach;

Breads, Grains, Cereals, Pasta

Danish pastry; Sweet rolls; Donuts; Muffins (blueberry); Muffins (oat bran); Croissant; Granola bars; Muffins (corn); Cereal (granola); Muffins (wheat bran); Cereal (wheat germ); Noodles (Chinese chow Mein); Bread (banana); Bread sticks; Crackers (wheat); Bread (cornbread); Noodles (egg); Biscuits; Waffles; Wheat germ; Crackers (milk); Corn; Barley; Rolls (whole-wheat dinner); Melba toast; Cereal (bran flakes); Crackers (whole-wheat);

Instead choose: Bread (white); Bread (pumpernickel); Couscous; Bread (whole-wheat); Crackers (saltines); Pasta; Spaghetti (spinach); Cereal (raisin bran); Popcorn (air popped); Oat bran; Rice (brown); Noodles (Japanese); Noodles (rice); Millet;

Dairy Products, Fats & Oils

Milk (chocolate); Hydrogenated vegetable oil; Vegetable shortening; Margarine; Oils: Ucuhuba Butter, palm, Cocoa Butter, Cupu Assu; Fat (duck, chicken & turkey); Lard; Cheese (American); Oils: cottonseed, tea seed; Butter; Other Oils; Margarine-like spreads; Non-dairy creamers; Cheese (Limburger); Cheese made w/whole milk; Fat (beef/lamb/pork); Various Cheese; Cheese spread; Cream (whipped); Milk (whole); Oils: hazelnut, safflower, canola; Cheese (Ricotta); Sour cream; Milk (2% fat); Buttermilk;

Instead choose: Milk (skim);

Desserts, Snacks, Beverages

Cake (chocolate); Chocolate mousse; Coffee liqueur; Cookies (chocolate chip); Cream puffs/Éclair; Crème de menthe; Ice cream (chocolate); Peanut butter; Puff pastry; Carob (candy); Dessert toppings; Molasses; Candies (peanut bar); Brownies; After-dinner mints; Cheesecake; Pies (various types); Chewing gum; Chocolate (sweet); Candies (peanut brittle); Candies (sesame crunch); Coffeecake; Halvah (candy); Pie (pumpkin); Chocolate (dark); Pie (coconut cream); Candies (caramel); Frostings; Sherbet; Candies (hard); Jams & Preserves; Jellies; Marshmallows; Cookies (butter); Cakes; Pie (vanilla cream); Pie (fried, fruit); Pie (lemon meringue); Pudding; Applesauce; Piña colada; Fruit leather/rolls; Ice cream (vanilla); Cookies; Soft (carbonated) drinks; Ice cream cones; Hot chocolate; Pie (apple); Pie (pecan); Honey; Frozen yogurt; Eggnog; Ginger ale; Taro chips; Beer; 80+ proof distilled alc. bev.; Fruit punch; Lemonade; Whiskey; Tonic water; Potato sticks; Milk shakes; Pancakes; Sports drinks; Red Bull (drink); Pie crust; Tortilla chips; Popcorn (oil popped); Potato chips; Malted drinks (nonalcoholic); Wine (red); Wine (white);

Instead choose: Soy milk; Popcorn (air popped); Tea (herbal); Tea (plain);

Herbs & Spices, Fast Foods, Prepared Foods

Foie gras or liver pate; **Syrup (chocolate)**; **Hot dog**; **Teriyaki sauce**; **Salad dressings**; **Syrups**; **Tahini**; **Tofu (fried)**; **Sugar (brown)**; **Sugar (table, powder)**; **Soy sauce**; **Chicken Nuggets**; **Barbecue sauce**; **French toast**; **Cheeseburger**; Breaded shrimp; Beef & Chicken broth & stock; Sausage (meatless); Hamburger; Tempeh; Natto; Nachos; Pickle (sweet); Potato salad; Hush puppies; Onion rings; Pizza; Hummus; Mayonnaise; Soup (beef barley); Gravies (canned); Hash brown potatoes; Cottonseed meal; Soup (chicken noodle); Soup (veg/beef); Taco shells; Ketchup; Potato pancakes; Miso; Sauce (Hoisin); Fish stock; French fries; Egg rolls (veg); Corn cakes; Falafel; Sugar (maple); Poppy seed; Cocoa;

Instead <u>*choose*</u>*: Dill weed; Sage; Sauerkraut; Balsamic vinegar; Various Herbs & Spices; Horseradish; Mustard; Pickles; Sauces; Tomato paste; Vinegar; Soup (clam chowder); Cole slaw;*

Alternative Therapies & Miscellaneous

Excess body weight; **Deep Fried Food**; **2+ alcoholic drinks/day**; **Corn syrup**; **Fasting (for a specific period; do not skip meals)**; Smoking/Tobacco; Aspirin; Smoked fish/foods; High dosages of Niacin; Prescription drugs (diuretics such as thiazide);

Key Nutrients & Herbal Meds

Trans fatty acids; **Alcohol**; **Brewer's Yeast**; **Fat (saturated)**; **Sugar (refined)**; Omega-6 fatty acid (LA); Purine; Sugar (fructose);

Diabetes Type 2 (& Gout)

Diabetes is a disorder that refers to our body's inability to use or convert food to the fuel needed by our cells.

Insulin is a hormone that helps the glucose (sugar) get into the body cells. In diabetes, the body is unable to create or properly use insulin. Without insulin, glucose stays in the blood and eventually makes its way to the urine, instead of serving as fuel to our muscles, tissues and brain.

There are different types of diabetes but the most common one is Diabetes Type 2 which represents 90-95% of diabetes cases, and is the focus of this section.

You are at most risk to develop diabetes Type 2 if you are obese. Your risk increases as you get older, if you are a member of a US minority group, are physically inactive, have a family history of the disease, have high blood pressure, have low level of good cholesterol, or have a high level of triglycerides.

Over time, excessive blood sugar level can cause serious health problems, in particular heart related issues. Over 65% of those with diabetes die from heart disease or stroke.

While there is no cure for diabetes type 2, there are numerous tools such as nutrition and exercise to help with the management of this disorder. In addition to managing the blood sugar level, the goal of diabetes management includes control of blood pressure, and cholesterol levels.

Choose these for Gout & Diabetes (Type 2)

Top 5 items to consume:

Various Cereals; Peppers; Red Cabbage & Green Leafy Vegetables; Yam, Tomatoes & Squash; Guava, Persimmons & Berries; & Exercise;

Food items and actions that could improve your health (within a food group, most helpful items are listed first):

Meat, Fish & Poultry

Surimi; Bass (seabass); Bluefish; Catfish; Drum; Mackerel (king); Marlin; Shark; Snapper; Spot; Sturgeon; Swordfish; Wolffish; Tilefish; Sucker; Mullet; Cisco; Tilapia; Cusk; Shad; Crab (Alaskan King); Grouper; Ling; Smelt; Whiting; Sablefish; Milkfish; Pollock; Bass (striped); Bass (freshwater); Rockfish; Oysters; Burbot; Lingcod; Pumpkinseed sunfish; Seatrout; Pout; Monkfish; Scup; Yellowtail; Pompano fish; Sheepshead; Lobster (spiny); Butterfish; Beef round steak; Dolphinfish (Mahi-Mahi); Eel; Turkey liver; Orange roughy; Chicken breast (no skin); White fish; Turbot; Conch; Beef filet mignon; Flatfish (flounder & sole); Octopus; Crab (Dungeness); Carp; Halibut; Salmon (pink); Trout; Tuna (blue fin); Tuna (canned); Tuna (yellowfin); Beef rib eye; Beef tenderloin/T-bone/porterhouse; Crab (snow); Bear meat; Croaker; Chicken liver; Clams; Snail; Pork liver; Cod; Veal shank; Beef top sirloin;

Eggs, Beans, Nuts and Seeds

Almonds; Seeds: chia, flaxseed; Hazelnuts or Filberts; Pecans; Peas (sugar/snap); Walnuts; Beans: hyacinth, navy, yardlong; Seeds (sunflower); Peas (green); Beans (fava); Chickpeas; Pine nuts; Other Beans; Black-eyed peas; Walnuts (black); Soybeans (green); Macadamia nuts; Pistachio nuts; Egg white; Peas (split); Seeds: safflower, sesame, watermelon; Pigeon peas; Other Seeds; Hickory nuts; Beechnuts; Soybeans (dried); Peanuts; Acorns; Butternuts; Egg yolk; Lupin; Cornnuts; Alfalfa sprouts; Soy milk;

Fruits & Juices

Guava; Persimmons; Cranberries; Grapefruit; Acerola; Blackberries; Raspberries; Kumquats; Avocado; Currants (raw); Lemon; Other Berries; Pitanga; Jujube (fruit); Rhubarb; Mango; Cherries (especially tart and including juice); Plantains; Rowal; Pumelo (Shaddock); Papaya; Orange juice; Abiyuch; Oranges; Cranberry juice; Grapefruit juice; Nectarine; Cantaloupe; Durian; Lime; Starfruit; Natal Plum (Carissa); Peaches; Plum; Pomegranate; Apples; Passion fruit; Kiwi fruit; Olives; Apricots; Tangerines; Apricots (dried); Peaches (dried); Pineapple juice; Litchi; Pineapple; Litchi (dried); Watermelon; Tamarind; Longans; Prunes (dried); Apple juice; Apples (dried); Dried fruits; Breadfruit; Banana; Pears; Figs; Honeydew melon; Grape juice; Pomegranate juice; Quince; Prune juice; Dates; Grapes; ***Avoid fruit juices made from concentrate or with added sugar***

Vegetables

Peppers (hot chili, red); Cabbage (red); Balsam pear leafy tips; Garden cress; Lambsquarters; Mustard spinach; Peppers (banana); Peppers; Pokeberry shoots; Taro (Tahitian); Taro leaves; Vine spinach (Basella); Cabbage (green); Yam; Amaranth leaves; Watercress; Winged beans leaves; Cabbage (savoy); Borage; Dandelion Greens; Tomatoes; Squash (Acorn); Bell peppers (red); Beet greens; Parsnips; Pumpkin flowers; Squash (Butternut); Sweet potatoes; Swiss chard; Kohlrabi; Cowpeas leafy tips; Chicory greens; Okra; Purslane; Turnip greens; Tomato juice; Bell peppers (green); Arugula; Broccoli; Celtuce; Green onions (scallions); Bok choy; Potatoes w/skin; Carrots; Chrysanthemum (Garland); Chrysanthemum Leaves; Endive; Grape leaves; Various Lettuce; Mushrooms (Chanterelle); Squash (Hubbard); Sweet potatoes leaves; Potato; Brussels sprouts; Sesbania Flower; Broccoli (Chinese); Epazote; Zucchini; Celery; Mustard greens; Lotus root; Kale; Cloud ear fungus; Mushrooms (Morel); Collards; Kelp; Mushrooms (shitake); Nopal; Taro; Balsam pear; Radishes; Fiddlehead ferns; Cauliflower; Arrowhead; Hearts of palm; Mushrooms (portabella); Leeks; Green beans; Shallots; Fennel (Bulb); Arrowroot; Spinach; Mushrooms (Jew's ear); Tomatoes (sun-dried); Cucumber with peel; Squash (Spaghetti); Wasabi root; Eggplant; Onions; Rutabaga; Turnips; Pumpkin; Artichoke (Jerusalem); Asparagus; Garlic; Beets; Artichoke;

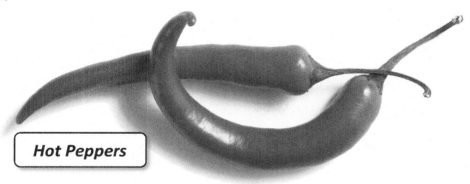

Hot Peppers

Breads, Grains, Cereals, Pasta

Cereal (shredded wheat); Cereal (corn flakes); Cereal (rice crisps); English muffins (whole-wheat); Cereals; Buckwheat; Tortillas (corn); Spaghetti (whole-wheat); Bread (wheat germ); Rice (wild); Rolls (whole-wheat dinner); Spelt; Oatmeal (cereal); Quinoa; Bread (pumpernickel); Bulgur; Bread (Italian); Rye grain; Toasted bread; English muffins; Noodles (Chinese chow Mein); Bagels; Whole-wheat; Triticale; Bread (French/Sourdough); Rice bran; Durum wheat; Rolls (French); Spaghetti; Amaranth; Biscuits; Corn bran; Crackers (whole-wheat); Bread (banana); Bread sticks; Bread (whole-grain); Bread (oat bran); Pasta; Sorghum grain; Wheat germ; Rice cakes (Brown rice); Wheat; Rice (brown); Cereal (granola); Oats; Millet; Rolls (Kaiser); Melba toast; Crackers (saltines); Semolina; Couscous; Waffles; Rolls (hamburger/hot dog); Barley;

Dairy Products, Fats & Oils

Cheese (Cottage); **Choose low-fat products**; Oil (wheat germ); Milk (1% fat); Fish oil (cod liver); Oils: flaxseed, safflower; Milk (skim); Oils: hazelnut, almonds; Buttermilk; Other Oils; Cream; Yogurt; Milk (2% fat); Milk (whole); Cheese (Parmesan); Cheese (Edam); Cheese (Gruyere); Other Cheese; Whey (sweet); Fish oil (salmon);

Desserts, Snacks, Beverages

Popcorn (air popped); **Potato chips**; **Popcorn (oil popped)**; **Tortilla chips**; **Water**; **Coffee (lowers Diabetes risk and Gout risk among men, decaf in particular)**; **Coffee (decaf)**; Pretzels; Pie crust; Potato sticks; Taro chips;

Herbs & Spices, Fast Foods, Prepared Foods

Cornmeal (whole-grain); **Egg rolls (veg)**; **Parsley**; **Tofu**; **Thyme (fresh)**; **Corn salad**; Cottonseed meal; Soup (minestrone); Soup (vegetable); French fries; Coriander/Cilantro; Basil (fresh); Taco shells; Hash brown potatoes; Dill weed; Potato pancakes; Cinnamon (Specially effective with pre-diabetic & D2 diabetic); Natto; Falafel; Soup (veg/beef); Cayenne (red) pepper; Rosemary (fresh); Spearmint (fresh); Tahini; Sage; Croutons; Macaroni; Succotash; Peppermint; Kimchi; Onion rings; Hummus; Mints; Tomato paste; Sauerkraut; Pepper (black);

Alternative Therapies & Miscellaneous

For diabetes, maintain annual physical exam; get vaccinated; monitor eyes, foot, blood pressure; Exercise (including cardiovascular, weight training, walking and jogging); **Fluids/juices/water**; Eat smaller more frequent meals; Glucomannan; Organically grown foods; Exposure to sun;

Key Nutrients & Herbal Meds

Starch/complex carbohydrates (Keep the total carb intake per meal constant); Goji berry; Celery seed; Chromium; Fat (monounsaturated); Fat (polyunsaturated); Fiber; Ginseng (Siberian); Gymnema; Psyllium; Vitamin A; Zinc; Beta Carotene; Vitamin C;

Do not choose these for Gout & Diabetes (Type 2)

Top 5 items to avoid:

Excess Body Weight; Fasting; Chocolate; Processed (luncheon) meats; Sweets; 2+ Alcoholic drinks/day;

Avoid or consume much less of the following (within a food group, most harmful items are listed first):

Meat, Fish & Poultry

Salami; **Bologna**; **Frankfurters**; **Luncheon meats**; **Pastrami**; **Pepperoni**; **Sausages**; **Chicken & Turkey skins**; **Chorizo**; **Beef jerky sticks**; **Beef tongue**; **Corned beef**; **Bacon**; **Beef kidneys**; **Lamb brain**; **Pork skins**; **Cured meats**; **Organ Meats**; **Lamb ribs**; **Fish roe**; Pork ribs; Caviar; Pork cured/ham; Squid (Calamari); Goose; Shrimp; Scallops; Beef (cured dried); Lamb; Pork; Rabbit meat; Duck (no skin); Venison; Veal loin; Beaver meat; Lobster; Crayfish; Frog legs; Quail breast; Guinea hen; Bison/buffalo meat; Veal shoulder; Turkey breast; Quail; Beef; Boar meat; Turkey dark meat; Abalone; Veal; Squab (pigeon);

Instead Choose: Chicken wings; Haddock; Northern pike; Whelk; Perch; Cisco (smoked); White fish (smoked); Mussels; Goat meat; Pork Loin; Beef Shank; Salmon (smoked, Lox); Anchovy; Herring; Mackerel; Sardines; Walleye; Crab (Blue); Beef ribs; Chicken dark meat (skinless); Cuttlefish;

Eggs, Beans, Nuts and Seeds

Coconut meat (dried); Coconut meat (raw); Coconut milk; Pili nuts; Egg (raw); Egg (hard-boiled); Cashew nuts; Lentils; Breadfruit seeds;

Instead Choose: Brazil nuts; Ginkgo nuts; Beans (lima);

Breads, Grains, Cereals, Pasta

Danish pastry; **Sweet rolls**; **Donuts**; **Muffins (blueberry)**; **Croissant**; Cereal (bran flakes); Muffins (corn); Crackers (wheat); Noodles (egg); Bread (white); Muffins (oat bran); Granola bars; Crackers (milk); Wheat bran;

Instead Choose: Spaghetti (spinach); Oat bran; Noodles (Japanese); Corn; Matzo crackers; Wheat bran muffins; Rice noodles; Cornbread; White rice;

Dairy Products, Fats & Oils

Hydrogenated vegetable oil; **Milk (chocolate)**; **Vegetable shortening**; **Oils: coconut, Ucuhuba Butter, Babassu**; **Margarine**; **Fat (beef/lamb/pork)**; **Fat (duck, chicken, turkey)**; **Lard**; **Oils: Cocoa Butter, Cupu Assu**; **Non-dairy creamers**; Oils: palm, Shea nut, tea seed, cottonseed; Cream (whipped); Butter; Cheese (American); Fish oil (menhaden); Margarine-like spreads; Fish oil (herring); Sour cream;

Instead Choose: Oil (peanut); Cheeses: Mozzarella, Brie, Roquefort, Cream, Romano, Limburger, Feta; Other Oils; Cheese spread; Fish Oil (Sardine);

Desserts, Snacks, Beverages

Applesauce; Cake (chocolate); Chocolate (dark or sweet); Chocolate mousse; Coffee liqueur; Cookies (chocolate chip); Cream puffs/Éclair; Crème de menthe; Hot chocolate; Ice cream (chocolate); Soft (carbonated) drinks; Puff pastry; Carob (candy); Dessert toppings; Red Bull (drink); Molasses; Brownies; Ginger ale; After-dinner mints; Cheesecake; Chewing gum; Piña colada; Fruit punch; Lemonade; Candies (peanut brittle); Eggnog; Candies (peanut bar); Coffeecake; Pie (coconut cream); Candies; Frostings; Jams & Preserves; Jellies; Marshmallows; Pudding; Sherbet; Cookies (butter); Tonic water; Cake (gingerbread); Pie (vanilla cream); Cakes; Pie (fried, fruit); Pie (lemon meringue); Sports drinks; Fruit leather/rolls; Ice cream (vanilla); Cookies; Halvah (candy); Ice cream cones; Frozen yogurt; Pie (pecan); Honey; Pie (apple); Milk shakes; Pancakes; 80+ proof distilled alc. bev.; Whiskey; Beer; Pie (pumpkin); Malted drinks (nonalcoholic); Candies (sesame crunch); Peanut butter; Tea (plain);

Instead _Choose_: Tea (herbal); Tea (green); Wine (red); Wine (white);

Herbs & Spices, Fast Foods, Prepared Foods

Syrup (chocolate); Teriyaki sauce; Hot dog; Barbecue sauce; Sugar (brown); Sugar (table, powder); Syrups; Salad dressings; Pickle (sweet); Soy sauce; Sauce (Hoisin); Ketchup; Miso; Chicken Nuggets; Chicken & Beef broth/stock; Gravies (canned); Pizza; Fish stock; Nachos; Foie gras or liver pate; Soup (chicken noodle); Cheeseburger; Sauces; Tabasco sauce; French toast; Sugar (maple); Tempeh; Breaded shrimp; Tofu (fried); Hamburger; Soup (clam chowder); Potato salad; Mayonnaise; Soup (beef barley); Hush puppies;

Instead _Choose_: Cole slaw; Sausage (meatless); Corn cakes; Cocoa; Balsamic vinegar; Capers; Herbs & Spices; Horseradish; Mustard; Pickles; Salt; Vinegar;

Alternative Therapies & Miscellaneous

2+ alcoholic drinks/day; Excess body weight; Fasting for a specific period (do not skip meals); Corn syrup; Deep-fried foods; Smoking/Tobacco; Prescription drugs (diuretics such as thiazide); Artificial sweeteners; Baking using butter; Abrupt changes in diet/exercise; Aspirin; Smoked fish/foods; High dosages of Niacin; Stress; Saccharine (NutraSweet); Processed or Refined foods; Aspartame (Equal);

Key Nutrients & Herbal Meds

Sugar (refined); Fat (saturated); Alcohol; Trans fatty acids; Cholesterol; Purine; Sugar (fructose); Sugar (total); Caffeine;

Obesity or Excess Body Weight (& Gout)

Obesity is defined as having too much body fat. It normally occurs when you continue to eat more calories than your body burns through exercise and normal daily activities. The unused calories are then stored as fat in your body leading to obesity.

Obesity is a risk factor for many diseases and illnesses including certain types of cancer. However, even a modest reduction in body fat (5 to 10% weight loss) can reduce your risk or delay illnesses caused by obesity.

The common way to measure obesity is body mass index (BMI). BMI is calculated by multiplying your weight in pounds by 703, divided by the square of your height in inches. For example a 6 feet tall man who weighs 190 pounds, has a BMI of 25.8. In the metric system, BMI is your weight in kilograms divided by the square of your height in meters.

Your BMI is considered normal if it is between 18.5 and 24.9. You are obese if your BMI is 30 or higher. You have excess body weight if your BMI is between 24.9 and 30.

Risk factors that can lead to obesity include: lack of physical exercise, overeating (e.g., oversized portions, recovery from quitting smoking), poor diet (e.g., eating high-fat foods), genetic or family history, pregnancy (inability to lose weight after giving birth), hormone problems, certain medications and illnesses, emotional issues (boredom, anger or stress), growing older, and lack of sleep.

Choose these for   Gout & Excess body weight

Top 5 items to consume:

Yam & Leafy Vegetables; Berries, Currants & Guava; Peppers; Squash & Potatoes; ... and Exercise

Food items and actions that could improve your health (within a food group, most helpful items are listed first):

Meat, Fish & Poultry (5.5 oz. of meat/fowl/fish or beans per day)

Surimi; Bass: freshwater, seabass, striped; Bluefish; Cisco; Drum; Mackerel (king); Marlin; Pollock; Smelt; Snapper; Spot; Sturgeon; Sucker; Swordfish; Tilefish; Whiting; Wolffish; Seatrout; Grouper; Tilapia; Burbot; Lingcod; Rockfish; Mullet; Cusk; Sheepshead; Ling; Catfish; Milkfish; Scup; Sablefish; Dolphinfish (Mahi-Mahi); Yellowtail; Pumpkinseed sunfish; Monkfish; Pout; Orange roughy; Butterfish; White fish; Turbot; Shad; Pompano fish; Salmon (pink); Trout; Tuna (blue fin); Tuna (yellowfin); Halibut; Cod; Walleye; Flatfish (flounder & sole); Shark;

Eggs, Beans, Nuts and Seeds (5.5 oz. of meat/fowl/fish or beans per day)

Beans: navy, yardlong, fava, hyacinth, yellow; Peas: sugar/snap, green; Seeds (chia); Other Beans; Lentils; Seeds (flaxseed); Black-eyed peas; Chickpeas; Peas (split); Pigeon peas; Alfalfa sprouts; Beans (kidney); Lupin;

Fruits & Juices (2 cups of fruits & juices per day)

Cranberries; Blackberries; Raspberries; Currants (raw); Guava; Lemon; Other Berries; Rhubarb; Cherries (especially tart, including juice); Oranges; Acerola; Kumquats; Pumelo (Shaddock); Persimmons; Abiyuch; Jujube (fruit); Lime; Starfruit; Kiwi fruit; Cranberry juice; Rowal; Grapefruit; Natal Plum (Carissa); Pomegranate; Pineapple; Nectarine; Papaya; Pitanga; Apples; Olives; Orange juice; Peaches; Plum; Durian; Litchi; Passion fruit; Breadfruit; Longans; Litchi (dried); Mango; Grapefruit juice; Tangerines; Currants (dried); Watermelon; Cantaloupe; Apples (dried); Dried fruits; Banana; Figs; Avocado; Honeydew melon; Pineapple juice; Plantains; Apricots; Pears; Quince; Apple juice; Grapes; Tamarind; Dates; Grape juice; Pomegranate juice; Raisins; **Avoid sugared or made from concentrate juices;**

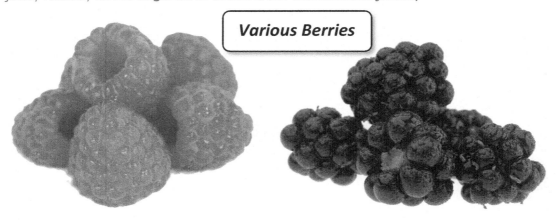

Various Berries

Vegetables (2.5 cups per day)

Yam; **Peppers (hot chili, red)**; **Balsam pear leafy tips**; **Taro leaves**; **Lambsquarters**; **Mustard spinach**; **Cabbage (red)**; **Peppers (pimento)**; **Peppers (banana)**; **Squash (Acorn)**; **Balsam pear**; **Cabbage (green)**; **Bell peppers (green)**; **Winged beans leaves**; **Parsnips**; **Cabbage (savoy)**; **Garden cress**; **Vine spinach (Basella)**; **Pokeberry shoots**; **Taro (Tahitian)**; **Grape leaves**; **Dandelion Greens**; **Potatoes w/skin**; **Peppers**; **Potato**; **Amaranth leaves**; **Squash (Butternut)**; **Sesbania Flower**; **Watercress**; **Celery**; **Kohlrabi**; **Broccoli**; **Turnip greens**; **Bell peppers (red)**; **Borage**; **Chicory greens**; **Cowpeas leafy tips**; **Sweet potatoes leaves**; **Beet greens**; **Carrots**; **Cloud ear fungus**; **Okra**; **Sweet potatoes**; **Pumpkin flowers**; **Tomatoes**; **Green onions (scallions)**; **Artichoke (Jerusalem)**; **Cucumber with peel**; **Chrysanthemum (Garland)**; **Chrysanthemum Leaves**; **Squash (Hubbard)**; **Swiss chard**; **Lotus root**; **Purslane**; **Endive**; **Bok choy**; **Brussels sprouts**; **Broccoli (Chinese)**; **Mushrooms (Chanterelle)**; **Arugula**; **Celtuce**; **Epazote**; **Mustard greens**; **Fiddlehead ferns**; **Fennel (Bulb)**; **Onions**; **Lettuce (loose leaf & Romaine)**; Taro; Tomatoes (sun-dried); Arrowroot; Lettuce (head); Nopal; Squash (Spaghetti); Wasabi root; Shallots; Collards; Kale; Eggplant; Zucchini; Artichoke; Radishes; Arrowhead; Beets; Kelp; Tomato juice; Mushrooms; Hearts of palm; Garlic; Pumpkin; Green beans; Turnips; Spinach; Rutabaga; Cauliflower; Leeks; Asparagus;

Breads, Grains, Cereals, Pasta (6 oz. of grains/day; 3+ oz. from whole grains)

Quinoa; Buckwheat; Tortillas (corn); Cereal (shredded wheat); Corn bran; Triticale; Rye grain; Amaranth; Oatmeal (cereal); Rice (brown); Rice (wild); Spaghetti (whole-wheat); Pasta; Sorghum grain; English muffins (whole-wheat); Cereal (cream of wheat); Bread (pumpernickel); Spelt;

Dairy Products, Fats & Oils (3 cups of low fat products per day)

Yogurt; Cheese (Cottage); Fish oil (salmon);

Desserts, Snacks, Beverages

Water; Popcorn (air popped); Coffee (decaf; lowers Gout risk for men); Tea (green); Coffee;

Herbs & Spices, Fast Foods, Prepared Foods

Cornmeal (whole-grain); Cayenne (red) pepper; Cinnamon; Parsley; Thyme (fresh); Tofu; Soup (minestrone); Soup (vegetable); Corn salad; Soup (tomato);

Alternative Therapies & Miscellaneous

Exercise (including cardiovascular, weight training, walking or jogging); Fluids/juices/water; Choose smaller food portions; Eat breakfast; Fat-free or low fat products; Weigh yourself daily; Organic cold-pressed oils; Wild fish and free range animals;

Key Nutrients & Herbal Meds

Starch/complex carbohydrates; Celery seed; Fiber; Omega-3 fatty acids; Psyllium; Vitamin C;

Do not choose these for   Gout & Excess body weight

Top 5 items to avoid:

>Cured & Processed (luncheon) Meats; Chocolate;
>Peanut Butter; Sweets; 2+ alcoholic drinks/day;

Avoid or consume much less of the following (within a food group, most harmful items are listed first):

Meat, Fish & Poultry

Bacon; **Cured Meats**; **Beef jerky sticks**; **Beef tongue**; **Beerwurst beer salami**; **Bologna (various)**; **Chorizo**; **Corned beef**; **Frankfurters**; **Luncheon meats**; **Pastrami**; **Pepperoni**; **Pork cured/ham**; **Pork liver cheese**; **Pork ribs**; **Salami**; **Sausages**; **Chicken skin**; **Lamb ribs**; **Pork shoulder**; **Beef (ground)**; **Beef chuck/brisket**; **Pork**; **Turkey skins**; **Organ Meats**; **Pork skins**; **Lamb**; **Beef**; **Goose**; **Lamb**; **Bison/buffalo meat**; **Veal**; **Game Meat**; **Rabbit meat**; **Venison**; **Quail**; Chicken dark meat; Chicken wings; Scallops; Squab (pigeon); Beef filet mignon; Goat meat; Shrimp; Frog legs; Duck (no skin); Abalone; Fish roe; Squid (Calamari); Sardines; Pheasant; Eel; Salmon (smoked, Lox); White fish (smoked); Lobster; Caviar; Turkey dark meat; Guinea hen; Quail breast; Whelk; Pheasant breast; Croaker; Cuttlefish; Crab (Blue); Crayfish; Clams; Tuna (canned); Snail; Turkey breast; Crab (Alaskan King); Anchovy; Octopus; Mussels;

Instead Choose: Northern pike; Perch; Haddock; Carp; Oysters; Spiny lobster; Dungeness Crab; Herring; Chicken breast (skinless); Mackerel; Conch; Snow crab; Cisco (smoked);

Eggs, Beans, Nuts and Seeds

Egg yolk; **Pili nuts**; **Cashew nuts**; **Brazil nuts**; **Coconut meat (dried)**; Peanuts; Butternuts; Hickory nuts; Soybeans (dried); Seeds (watermelon); Pine nuts; Seeds (pumpkin/squash); Coconut meat (raw); Seeds: cottonseed, sunflower, sesame, safflower; Beechnuts; Pecans; Walnuts (black); Coconut milk; Walnuts; Almonds; Acorns; Pistachio nuts; Hazelnuts or Filberts; Egg (duck); Egg (hard-boiled); Egg (raw); Soy milk; Macadamia nuts; Soybeans (green); Chestnuts; Ginkgo nuts; Cornnuts; Breadfruit seeds;

Instead Choose: Seeds (breadnut tree); Beans (lima); Egg substitute; Beans (baked); Egg white;

Breads, Grains, Cereals, Pasta

Sweet rolls; **Danish pastry**; **Donuts**; **Muffins (blueberry)**; **Muffins (oat bran)**; **Croissant**; **Wheat germ**; **Granola bars**; Noodles (Chinese chow Mein); Cereal (granola); Muffins: corn, wheat bran; Bread sticks; Melba toast; Cereal (wheat germ); Crackers (wheat); Cereal (bran flakes); Bread (banana); Crackers (milk); Bread (cornbread); Rice cakes (Brown rice); Rolls (hamburger/hot dog); Biscuits; Waffles; Rolls (whole-wheat dinner); Noodles (egg); Cereal (raisin bran); Corn; Wheat; Rolls (Kaiser); Bread (wheat germ); Whole-wheat; Couscous; Crackers (whole-wheat); Toasted bread; Bread (white); Bread (oat bran); Rice (white); Crackers (matzo); Crackers (saltines); Wheat bran;

Instead Choose: Cereal (whole-wheat); Oat bran; Oats; English muffins; Spaghetti; Bulgur; other Bread; other cereals; Millet; Bagels; other Noodles; Rice bran; Durum wheat; Barley; Spinach spaghetti; Semolina;

Dairy Products, Fats & Oils

Milk (chocolate); **Hydrogenated vegetable oil**; **Vegetable shortening**; **Margarine**; **Oils: Ucuhuba Butter, palm, Babassu, coconut, Cocoa Butter, Cupu Assu**; **Fat (duck)**; **Lard**; **Cheese (American)**; **Oil (cottonseed)**; **Butter**; **Fat (chicken & turkey)**; **Oils: tea seed, wheat germ, corn, poppy seed, sesame, tomato seeds**; **Margarine-like spreads**; **Non-dairy creamers**; **Cheese (Limburger)**; Fat (beef/lamb/pork); other Oils; other Cheese; Cheese spread; Cream (whipped); Sour cream; Cheese (Ricotta); Oil (canola); Milk (2% fat); Milk (whole); Oil (olive); Buttermilk; Fish oil (menhaden);

Instead _Choose_: *Oil (flaxseed); Fish oil (cod liver); Cream; Milk (1%); Sweet whey; other Fish oil; Skim Milk;*

Desserts, Snacks, Beverages

Applesauce; **Cake (chocolate)**; **Chocolate (dark or sweet)**; **Chocolate mousse**; **Coffee liqueur**; **Cookies (chocolate chip)**; **Cream puffs/Éclair**; **Crème de menthe**; **Hot chocolate**; **Ice cream (chocolate)**; **Molasses**; **Peanut butter**; **Puff pastry**; **Carob (candy)**; **Dessert toppings**; **Red Bull (drink)**; **Candies (peanut bar)**; **Brownies**; **Ginger ale**; **After-dinner mints**; **Cheesecake**; **Chewing gum**; **Fruit punch**; **Lemonade**; **Candies**; **Coffeecake**; **Halvah (candy)**; **Pie (pumpkin)**; **Eggnog**; **Pie (coconut cream)**; **Frostings**; **Jams & Preserves**; **Jellies**; **Marshmallows**; **Sherbet**; **Soft (carbonated) drinks**; **Cookies**; **Tonic water**; **Cake (gingerbread)**; **Pie (vanilla cream)**; **Piña colada**; **Cake (pound)**; **Cakes**; **Pie (fried, fruit)**; **Various Pies**; **Fruit leather/rolls**; **Ice cream (vanilla)**; **Ice cream cones**; **Frozen yogurt**; **Honey**; **Pudding**; **Milk shakes**; **Pancakes**; **Taro chips**; **Beer**; Potato sticks; 80+ proof distilled alc. bev.; Whiskey; Sports drinks; Pie crust; Tortilla chips; Popcorn (oil popped); Pretzels; Malted drinks (nonalcoholic); Tea (plain)

Instead _Choose_: *Tea (herbal); Wine; Potato chips;*

Herbs & Spices, Fast Foods, Prepared Foods

Foie gras or liver pate; **Hot dog**; **Syrup (chocolate)**; **Teriyaki sauce**; **Barbecue sauce**; **Sugar (brown)**; **Sugar (table, powder)**; **Syrups**; **Soy sauce**; **Salad dressings**; **Chicken Nuggets**; **Tahini**; **Tofu (fried)**; **Pickle (sweet)**; **Ketchup**; **Sauce (Hoisin)**; **Beef broth & stock**; **Sausage (meatless)**; **Chicken broth & stock**; **French toast**; **Hamburger**; **Cheeseburger**; Corn cakes; Breaded shrimp; Tempeh; Nachos; Miso; Hush puppies; Onion rings; Pizza; Sauce (fish); Gravies (canned); Potato salad; Hash brown potatoes; Fish stock; Sauce (oyster); Taco shells; Hummus; Falafel; Sauce (Sofrito); Potato pancakes; Mayonnaise; Soup (beef barley); Sauces; Tabasco sauce; Cottonseed meal; Soup (chicken noodle); Salt (table); Soup (veg/beef); Cocoa; Natto; Sugar (maple); French fries; Cole slaw; Croutons; Poppy seed;

Instead _Choose_: *Rosemary (fresh); Dill weed; Succotash; Pepper (black); Sage; Macaroni; various herbs & spices; Tomato paste; Clam Chowder soup; Balsamic Vinegar; Horseradish; Pickle; Vinegar; Egg rolls (veg); Sauerkraut; Mustard; Kimchi; Capers;*

Alternative Therapies & Miscellaneous

2+ alcoholic drinks/day; **Corn syrup**; **Deep-fried foods**; **Smoked fish/foods**; **Excess body weight**; Tapioca pearls; Artificial sweeteners; Saccharine (NutraSweet); Aspartame (Equal); Aspirin; Excessive TV viewing (avoid eating while watching); Fasting (for a specific period; do not skip meals); Food additives/preservatives; High dosages of Niacin; Prescription drugs (diuretics such as thiazide); Processed or Refined foods; Stress;

Key Nutrients & Herbal Meds

Sugar (refined); **Trans fatty acids**; **Fat (saturated)**; Alcohol; Brewer's Yeast; Omega-6 fatty acid (LA); Purine; Sugar (fructose); Caffeine; **Limit calorie consumption per day to 10 per pound of desired weight**;

Depression (& Gout)

Depression is a serious chronic illness. It is not just a temporary feeling of being down. It is a disorder of the brain. It can interfere with your normal life and lead to various physical and emotional problems. It affects men, women and elderly in different ways.

The exact cause of depression is unknown. But several factors can lead to depression: loss of a loved one, stressful situations such as a difficult relationship or financial problems, family history of depression (genetic factors), differences in brain chemistry, changes in body hormones, and traumatic events during one's childhood.

You are more likely to get depression if you are between 15 and 30 years old, you are a woman, it is winter time, or it is just after you gave birth to a baby.

Choose these for Gout & Depression

Top 5 items to consume:

Corn Flakes/Cereals; Green Leafy Vegetables & Peppers; Currants, Cherries & Oranges; Juices & Water; Yam; ... and Exercise

Food items and actions that could improve your health (within a food group, most helpful items are listed first):

Meat, Fish & Poultry

Surimi; Various Bass; Bluefish; Burbot; Butterfish; Catfish; Cisco; Cusk; Dolphinfish (Mahi-Mahi); Drum; Grouper; Ling; Lingcod; Mackerel (king); Marlin; Milkfish; Mullet; Pollock; Pout; Pumpkinseed sunfish; Rockfish; Scup; Seatrout; Shad; Sheepshead; Smelt; Snapper; Spot; Sturgeon; Sucker; Swordfish; Tilapia; Tilefish; Turbot; Whiting; Wolffish; Yellowtail; Monkfish; Conch; Various Crabs; Cuttlefish; Octopus; Whelk; Lobster (spiny); Orange roughy; Clams; Shark; Pompano fish; Sablefish; Turkey breast; Turkey dark meat; Turkey liver; Cod; Flatfish (flounder & sole); Haddock; Mussels; White fish; Beef spleen; Oysters; Chicken breast (no skin); Turkey giblets; Caribou meat; Carp; Halibut; Northern pike; Perch; Salmon (pink); Trout; Tuna (blue fin); Tuna (yellowfin); Walleye; Crayfish; Croaker; Snail; Chicken giblets; Chicken liver; Pork liver; Veal shank;

Eggs, Beans, Nuts and Seeds

Seeds (flaxseed); Egg (duck); Peas (sugar/snap); Egg white; Seeds (chia); Beans: navy, fava; Seeds (breadnut tree); Egg (hard-boiled); Beans: hyacinth, yardlong; Egg (raw); Peas (green); Chickpeas; Egg yolk; Ginkgo nuts; Other Beans; Black-eyed peas; Breadfruit seeds; Chestnuts; Macadamia nuts; Lentils; Cornnuts; Pigeon peas; Soybeans (green); Egg substitute; Lupin; Acorns; Soybeans (dried); Seeds: cottonseed, safflower, sunflower; Almonds; Alfalfa sprouts; Peas (split); Hazelnuts or Filberts; Walnuts; Pistachio nuts;

Fruits & Juices

Orange juice; Currants (raw); Cherries (especially tart, including juice); Cranberry juice; Guava; Oranges; Cranberries; Acerola; Jujube (fruit); Lemon; Litchi; Longans; Persimmons; Pumelo (Shaddock); Grapefruit juice; Mulberries; Strawberries; Rhubarb; Various Berries; Kumquats; Litchi (dried); Pineapple; Abiyuch; Kiwi fruit; Papaya; Tamarind; Pomegranate; Natal Plum (Carissa); Grapefruit; Mango; Nectarine; Durian; Rowal; Currants (dried); Breadfruit; Lime; Starfruit; Pineapple juice; Peaches; Plum; Plantains; Olives; Pears (dried); Apples (dried); Apples; Apple juice; Pitanga; Tangerines; Avocado; Cantaloupe; Banana; Figs; Dried Fruits; Watermelon; Grape juice; Pomegranate juice; Prune juice; Passion fruit; Honeydew melon; Grapes; Quince; Dates; Pears; Apricots; Raisins; **Avoid sugared and made from concentrate juices;**

Vegetables

Peppers (hot chili, red); Balsam pear leafy tips; Garden cress; Lambsquarters; Mustard spinach; Peppers (hot chili); Peppers (pimento); Sesbania Flower; Taro leaves; Vine spinach (Basella); Taro (Tahitian); Amaranth leaves; Winged beans leaves; Cabbage (red); Balsam pear; Other Peppers; Pokeberry shoots; Cowpeas leafy tips; Yam; Dandelion Greens; Bell peppers (red); Cabbage (savoy); Turnip greens; Cabbage (green); Potatoes w/skin; Squash (Acorn); Kohlrabi; Broccoli; Watercress; Arrowroot; Epazote; Grape leaves; Kelp; Chrysanthemum (Garland); Chrysanthemum Leaves; Borage; Bok choy; Brussels sprouts; Okra; Bell peppers (green); Chicory greens; Beet greens; Pumpkin flowers; Swiss chard; Tomato juice; Arugula; Parsnips; Kale; Mustard greens; Endive; Lettuce (Romaine); Sweet potatoes; Garlic; Broccoli (Chinese); Lotus root; Collards; Purslane; Squash (Butternut); Sweet potatoes leaves; Potato; Beets; Celtuce; Green onions (scallions); Tomatoes; Celery; Arrowhead; Mushrooms (Chanterelle); Shallots; Tomatoes (sun-dried); Cauliflower; Onions; Spinach; Hearts of palm; Nopal; Squash (Hubbard); Taro; Artichoke (Jerusalem); Carrots; Cucumber with peel; Fennel (Bulb); Various Lettuce; other vegetables;

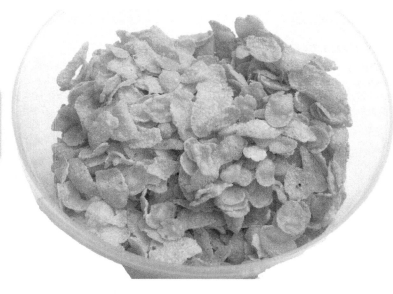

Corn Flakes & Other Cereals

Breads, Grains, Cereals, Pasta

Cereal (corn flakes); Cereal (rice crisps); English muffins (whole-wheat); Bread (French/Sourdough); Various Cereals; Bread (Italian); Toasted bread; Bread (whole-wheat); Buckwheat; Spaghetti (whole-wheat); Quinoa; Bread (wheat germ); Amaranth; Spelt; Bread (oat bran); Oatmeal (cereal); Triticale; Rice (wild); Bagels; English muffins; Whole-wheat; Bread (pumpernickel); Bulgur; Tortillas (corn); Cereal (wheat germ); Durum wheat; Rye grain; Rice (brown); Rolls (French); Oats; Spaghetti; Sorghum grain; Millet; Bread sticks; Rolls (Kaiser); Bread (white); Pasta; Rolls (hamburger/hot dog); Wheat bran; Rolls (whole-wheat dinner); Biscuits; Cereal (cream of wheat); Rice bran; Waffles; Barley; Crackers (whole-wheat); Rice (white); Bread (cornbread); Semolina; Wheat; Bread (banana); Melba toast; Couscous; Rice cakes (Brown rice);

Dairy Products, Fats & Oils

Cheese (Cottage); Low-fat products; Milk (1% fat); Fish oil (salmon); Milk (skim); Yogurt; Cream; Various Fish oil; Cheese (Brie); Whey (sweet); Cheese (Feta); Cheese (Romano); Cheese (Gjetost); Other Cheeses; Sour cream;

Desserts, Snacks, Beverages

Water (drink 8 cups of fluid per day); **Popcorn (air popped)**; **Pretzels**; Coffee (decaf; lowers Gout risk for men); Popcorn (oil popped); Potato chips; Coffee;

Herbs & Spices, Fast Foods, Prepared Foods

Cornmeal (whole-grain); **Tofu**; Cottonseed meal; Potato pancakes; Parsley; Corn salad; Egg rolls (veg); Thyme (fresh); Falafel; French fries; Croutons; Macaroni; Kimchi; Corn cakes; Hamburger; Taco shells; Succotash;

Alternative Therapies & Miscellaneous

Exercise (including cardiovascular, weight training, walking or jogging); Fluids/juices/water; Fresh (uncooked) fruits & vegetables; Socialize, join a club; Wild fish and free range animals; Organic cold-pressed oils;

Key Nutrients & Herbal Meds

Starch/complex carbohydrates; Celery seed; DHEA (dehydroepiandosterone); Folic Acid; Ginkgo Biloba; Omega-3 fatty acids; SAMe (works best with Vitamin B12 and Folic acid); St. John's wort (a dose of 2-4 grams of the herb for a mild antidepressant action or nervous disturbances); Valerian (don't combine with alcohol); Vitamin C;

Do not choose these for Gout & Depression

Top 5 items to avoid:

Chocolate; Alcoholic Beverages; Sweets & Corn Syrup; Luncheon (Processed) Meats; Salad Dressings;

Avoid or consume much less of the following (within a food group, most harmful items are listed first):

Meat, Fish & Poultry

Bologna; **Frankfurters**; **Pepperoni**; **Sausages**; **Salami**; **Bacon**; **Luncheon meats**; **Pastrami**; **Chorizo**; **Beef (cured brkfst strips)**; **Chicken & Turkey skins**; **Corned beef**; **Cured Meats**; **Pork cured/ham**; **Beef tongue**; **Pork liver cheese**; **Beef (cured dried)**; **Pork skins**; **Pork ribs**; **Goose**; Pork spare ribs; Beef (ground); Pork; Beef chuck/brisket; Lamb ribs; Beef; Quail; Chicken dark meat; Lamb tongue; Chicken wings; Fish roe; Squab (pigeon); Duck (no skin); Scallops; Guinea hen; Pheasant; Bison/buffalo meat; Veal shoulder; Organ Meats; Quail breast; Pheasant breast; Frog legs; Liver; Lamb; Veal loin; Boar meat; Abalone;

Instead <u>*Choose*</u>*: Squid (Calamari); Cisco (smoked); White fish (smoked); Eel; Beef round steak; Goat meat; Tuna (canned); Shrimp; Salmon (smoked, lox); Anchovy; Herring; Mackerel; Sardines; Lobster; Venison; Beef filet mignon; Caviar; Rabbit meat; Lamb leg; Pork loin/sirloin;*

Eggs, Beans, Nuts and Seeds

Coconut meat (dried); Coconut milk; Cashew nuts; Pili nuts; Soy milk;

Instead <u>*Choose*</u>*: Seeds (pumpkin/squash); Walnuts (black); Seeds (sesame); Pecans; Beechnuts; Watermelon seeds; Pine nuts; Hickory nuts; Coconut meat (raw); Peanuts; Brazil nuts; Butternuts;*

Breads, Grains, Cereals, Pasta

Danish pastry; **Sweet rolls**; **Donuts**; **Muffins (blueberry)**; **Granola bars**; Cereal (granola); Crackers (wheat); Muffins (oat bran); Crackers (milk); Noodles (egg); Croissant; Muffins (wheat bran);

Instead <u>*Choose*</u>*: Corn; Noodles (Chinese chow Mein); Crackers (saltines); Oat bran; Spaghetti (spinach); Wheat germ; other noodles; Matzo crackers; Corn Muffins;*

Dairy Products, Fats & Oils

Milk (chocolate); **Vegetable shortening**; **Hydrogenated vegetable oil**; **Margarine**; **Margarine-like spreads**; **Non-dairy creamers**; **Oil (cottonseed)**; Oils: corn, poppy seed, sesame, tomato seeds, tea seed; Fat (chicken, turkey, & duck); Lard; Oil (palm); Butter; Oil (Ucuhuba Butter); Cheese (American); Other oils; Fat (beef/lamb/pork); Oil (canola); Cheese (Cream); Cream (whipped); Oil (olive);

Instead <u>*Choose*</u>*: Cheese (Colby); Oil (flaxseed); Cheese (Ricotta); Milk (2% fat); Milk (whole); Cheese (Pimento); Cheese spread; Buttermilk; Cheese (Cheddar);*

Desserts, Snacks, Beverages

Cake (chocolate); Chocolate (sweet); Chocolate mousse; Coffee liqueur; Cookies (chocolate chip); Cream puffs/Éclair; Crème de menthe; Hot chocolate; Ice cream (chocolate); Puff pastry; Dessert toppings; Soft (carbonated) drinks; Candies (peanut bar); Brownies; Carob (candy); Cheesecake; After-dinner mints; Candies (peanut brittle); Coffeecake; Peanut butter; Chewing gum; Candies (caramel); Frostings; Pudding; Pie (coconut cream); Cookies (butter); Applesauce; Cake (gingerbread); Pie (vanilla cream); Pie (pumpkin); Cakes; Various Pies; Piña colada; Ginger ale; Halvah (candy); 80+ proof distilled alc. bev.; Fruit punch; Lemonade; Whiskey; Cookies; Jams & Preserves; Jellies; Sherbet; Marshmallows; Fruit leather/rolls; Candies; Ice cream (vanilla); Eggnog; Beer; Tonic water; Red Bull (drink); Taro chips; Molasses; Frozen yogurt; Honey; Sports drinks; Milk shakes; Potato sticks; Chocolate (dark); Pancakes; Wine (red); Wine (white); Tea (plain); Ice cream cones;

Instead <u>***Choose***</u>***: Malted drinks (nonalcoholic); Tea (herbal); Pie crust; Tortilla chips; Tea (green);***

Herbs & Spices, Fast Foods, Prepared Foods

Syrup (chocolate); Teriyaki sauce; Barbecue sauce; Sugar (table, powder); Salad dressings; Hot dog; Sugar (brown); Syrup (table blends); Chicken Nuggets; Ketchup; Pickle (sweet); Syrups; Soy sauce; Sauce (Hoisin); Nachos; Foie gras or liver pate; Onion rings; Chicken broth & stock; Pizza; Gravies (canned); Beef broth & stock; Breaded shrimp; Tahini; Sausage (meatless); Hush puppies; Fish stock; Mayonnaise; Soup (chicken noodle); Cocoa; Tofu (fried); Sauces; Tabasco sauce; Potato salad; Soup (beef barley); Sauce (fish); Miso; Soup (veg/beef); Hummus; French toast; Natto; Tempeh; Poppy seed; Hash brown potatoes;

Instead <u>***Choose***</u>***: Dill weed; Mints; Sauerkraut; Cole slaw; Soup (clam chowder); Sage; Cheeseburger; Balsamic vinegar; Herbs & Spices; Horseradish; Mustard; Black Pepper; Pickle; Salt; Maple sugar; Tomato paste; Vinegar; Hash brown potatoes;***

Alternative Therapies & Miscellaneous

2+ alcoholic drinks/day; Corn syrup; Excess body weight (avoid low carb diets); Deep-fried foods; Prescription drugs (diuretics such as thiazide); Fasting (for a specific period; don't skip meals); Smoking/Tobacco; Artificial sweeteners (e.g., sorbitol, mannitol, xylitol, maltitol and isomaltose); Aspirin; Smoked fish/foods; High dosages of Niacin; Processed or Refined foods; Saccharine (NutraSweet);

Key Nutrients & Herbal Meds

Alcohol; Sugar (refined); Brewer's Yeast; Trans fatty acids; Marijuana; Omega-6 fatty acid (LA); Purine; Sugar (fructose); Fat (saturated); Caffeine;

Alzheimer's Disease (& Gout)

Dementia is a brain disorder that refers to our loss of ability to think, remember, reason and perform daily activities. Among people older than 60, Alzheimer's Disease (AD) is the most common cause of dementia.

AD causes the gradual decline and loss of brain cells and the ability for cells (neuron) to communicate with each other. Thus a person affected with AD, has fewer brain cells and fewer connections among the brain's remaining cells. This results in a steady decline in our memory (as in remembering people's names, or doing daily tasks), and cognitive functions such as reasoning.

A combination of factors is believed to cause AD. Among these risk factors are: age (starting at the age of 60 and increasing over time), immediate family history of AD, sex (women are more likely than men to develop AD), and the same risk factors associated with heart disease (i.e., high blood pressure, high cholesterol, diabetes, lack of exercise and smoking). Higher levels of on-going intellectual and social activities have been found to reduce the risk of developing AD.

There is neither a proven approach to prevent nor to cure this disease. But there has been a 2015 study conducted by the scientists at the Rush University, whereby a combination of the Mediterranean diet and DASH (Dietary Approaches to Stop Hypertension) diet, known as the MIND diet, has shown that this diet can lower the risk of AD significantly. There has also been some evidence that reducing risk of high blood pressure, high cholesterol, obesity and diabetes can reduce the risk of developing AD. Therefore, proper nutrition, exercise and staying mentally and socially active can all play an important role.

Choose these for Gout & Alzheimer's Disease

Top 5 items to consume:

Peppers; Berries; Leafy Vegetables; Celery, Bell Peppers & Okra; Yam; and Exercise;

Food items and actions that could improve your health (within a food group, most helpful items are listed first):

Meat, Fish & Poultry

Surimi; Bass (freshwater, seabass, striped); Bluefish; Catfish; Drum; Marlin; Pollock; Smelt; Snapper; Spot; Sturgeon; Sucker; Swordfish; Tilefish; Whiting; Wolffish; Seatrout; Cisco; Rockfish; Mackerel (king); Mullet; Shad; Pompano fish; Sablefish; Burbot; Grouper; Lingcod; Tilapia; Ling; Dolphinfish (Mahi-Mahi); Sheepshead; Cusk; Milkfish; Pumpkinseed sunfish; Scup; Shark; White fish; Orange roughy; Yellowtail; Butterfish; Pout; Monkfish; Turbot; Fish (1+ servings/week for AD); Carp; Halibut; Salmon (pink); Trout; Tuna (blue fin); Walleye; Conch; Flatfish (flounder & sole); Perch; Eel;

Eggs, Beans, Nuts and Seeds

Macadamia nuts; Peas (sugar/snap); Nuts (5+ servings/week for AD); Hazelnuts or Filberts; Walnuts; Cornnuts; Chestnuts; Ginkgo nuts; Breadfruit seeds; Almonds; Pecans; Walnuts (black); Peas (green); Acorns; Beans (yardlong); Seeds (flaxseed); Pine nuts; Beans (hyacinth); Pistachio nuts; Beans (fava); Hickory nuts; Beechnuts; Seeds (chia); Beans (navy); Brazil nuts; Butternuts; Beans: moth beans, mung, adzuki, black, Great Northern); Egg white; Pili nuts; Lentils; Beans/Legumes (1+ servings every other day for AD);

Fruits & Juices

Cranberry juice; Cranberries; Various Berries (2+ servings/week for AD); Pomegranate; Orange juice; Currants (raw); Cherries (especially tart, including juice); Oranges; Acerola; Guava; Jujube (fruit); Lemon; Litchi; Longans; Persimmons; Pumelo (Shaddock); Grapefruit juice; Rhubarb; Kumquats; Litchi (dried); Pineapple; Abiyuch; Kiwi fruit; Papaya; Natal Plum (Carissa); Grapefruit; Nectarine; Tamarind; Rowal; Currants (dried); Breadfruit; Lime; Starfruit; Grapes; Pineapple juice; Peaches; Plum; Mango; Olives; Pears (dried); Apples; Apples (dried); Apple juice; Pitanga; Plantains; Tangerines; Dried fruits; Durian; Cantaloupe; Grape juice; Avocado; Figs; Watermelon; Pomegranate juice; Banana; Prune juice; Honeydew melon; Quince; Passion fruit; Dates; Pears; Apricots; **Avoid sugared or made from concentrate juices;**

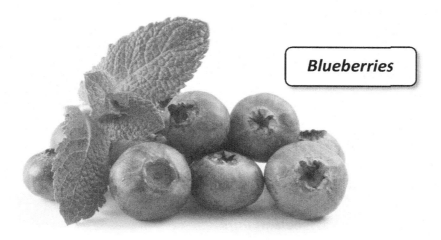

Blueberries

Vegetables (green leafy vegetables or a salad, and one other vegetable everyday)

Peppers (hot chili, red); Cabbage (red); Balsam pear leafy tips; Garden cress; Lambsquarters; Mustard spinach; Peppers; Taro leaves; Vine spinach (Basella); Taro (Tahitian); Cabbage (green); Amaranth leaves; Watercress; Winged beans leaves; Balsam pear; Pokeberry shoots; Sesbania Flower; Dandelion Greens; Beet greens; Swiss chard; Celery; Bell peppers (red); Kohlrabi; Chicory greens; Okra; Turnip greens; Cowpeas leafy tips; Borage; Bell peppers (green); Arugula; Broccoli; Fiddlehead ferns; Green onions (scallions); Yam; Cabbage (savoy); Epazote; Grape leaves; Various Lettuce; Sweet potatoes leaves; Squash (Acorn); Chrysanthemum Leaves; Potatoes w/skin; Brussels sprouts; Broccoli (Chinese); Pumpkin flowers; Bok choy; Tomato juice; Zucchini; Purslane; Mustard greens; Kale; Lotus root; Sweet potatoes; Tomatoes; Parsnips; Squash (Butternut); Mushrooms (Chanterelle); Collards; Celtuce; Kelp; Onions; Cucumber with peel; Garlic; Arrowhead; Nopal; Tomatoes (sun-dried); Shallots; Artichoke; Taro; Arrowroot; Chrysanthemum (Garland); Squash (Hubbard); Potato; Artichoke (Jerusalem); Beets; Carrots; Endive; Fennel (Bulb); Squash (Spaghetti); Wasabi root; Radishes; Cauliflower; Green beans; Spinach; Mushrooms; Hearts of palm; Eggplant; Rutabaga; Turnips; Pumpkin; Leeks; Asparagus

Breads, Grains, Cereals, Pasta

Cereal (whole-wheat); Buckwheat; Whole Grains (3+ servings/day); English muffins (whole-wheat); Spaghetti (whole-wheat); Amaranth; Quinoa; Triticale; Whole-wheat; Cereal (rice crisps); Spelt; Oatmeal (cereal); Bulgur; Durum wheat; Rye grain; Cereal (shredded wheat); Rice (wild); Cereal (corn flakes); Sorghum grain; Oats; Rice (brown); Bread (whole-wheat); Millet; Various Cereals; Tortillas (corn); Spaghetti; Bagels; Bread (French/Sourdough); English muffins; Wheat bran; Rice (white); Crackers (whole-wheat); Barley; Pasta; Semolina; Wheat; Bread (Italian); Bread (wheat germ); Rolls (whole-wheat dinner); Toasted bread; Bread (oat bran); Couscous; Corn;

Dairy Products, Fats & Oils

Fish oil (cod liver); Oil (olive); Various Fish oil; Milk (1% fat); Oil (flaxseed); Fat-free or low fat products; Milk (skim); Whey (sweet); Cream; Yogurt; Buttermilk;

Desserts, Snacks, Beverages

Popcorn (air popped); **Coffee (lowers risk of Gout for men, decaf in particular)**; **Water**; Wine (one glass of wine/day for AD); Coffee (decaf); Tea (green); Popcorn (oil popped); Potato chips; Tea (plain); Tortilla chips

Herbs & Spices, Fast Foods, Prepared Foods

Cornmeal (whole-grain); **Parsley**; Thyme (fresh); Turmeric; Tofu; Corn salad; Basil (fresh); Coriander/Cilantro; Mints; Peppermint; Rosemary (fresh); Spearmint (fresh); Macaroni; Cinnamon; Cocoa; Cole slaw; Croutons; Falafel;

Alternative Therapies & Miscellaneous

Exercise (i.e., Cardiovascular, Weight Training, walking, jogging, or cycling); **Fluids/Juices/Water**; Challenge your mind (puzzles, games, books); Mediterranean diet (can reduce risk of AD by 53%); Exposure to sun; Fresh (uncooked) fruits/veg's; Wild fish and free range animals; Green plants and vegetables;

Key Nutrients & Herbal Meds

Celery seed; Chlorophyll; Omega-3 fatty acids; Starch/complex carbohydrates; Vitamin C;

<u>*Do not*</u> choose these for Gout & Alzheimer's Disease

Top 5 items to avoid:

Bacon, Cured & Luncheon Meats; Sweets; Teriyaki & Soy Sauces; Hydrogenated Vegetable Oil; Red & Organ Meats; & Excess Body Weight;

Avoid or consume much less of the following (within a food group, most harmful items are listed first):

Meat, Fish & Poultry

Bacon; **Cured Meats**; **Salami**; **Bologna**; **Chorizo**; **Frankfurters**; **Luncheon meats**; **Pastrami**; **Pepperoni**; **Sausages**; **Pork cured/ham**; **Beef jerky sticks**; **Pork ribs**; **Corned beef**; **Lamb ribs**; **Beef tongue**; **Pork skins**; **Pork shoulder**; **Veal heart**; **Pork spare ribs**; **Beef (ground)**; **Pork**; **Beef chuck/brisket**; **Liver**; **Organ Meats**; **Lamb**; **Chicken skin**; **Bison/buffalo meat**; **Veal**; **Turkey skins**; **Beef**; **Meat (limit to 4 or less servings/week)**; **Game Meat**; **Rabbit meat**; **Venison**; **Goat meat**; Frog legs; Scallops; Goose; Shrimp; Fish roe; Abalone; Chicken dark meat; Quail; Chicken wings; Tuna (canned); Lobster; Squid (Calamari); Salmon (smoked, Lox); Duck (no skin); Caviar; Clams; Squab (pigeon); Quail breast; Pheasant; Crab (Blue); Sardines; Pheasant breast; Crab (Alaskan King); Cuttlefish; Crayfish; Guinea hen;

Instead <u>Choose</u>: Tuna (yellowfin); Cod; Oysters; Cisco (smoked); Snail; Turkey dark meat; Lobster spiny; Crab Dungeness; Northern pike; Chicken breast no skin; Haddock; Anchovy; Herring; Mackerel; Turkey breast; White fish smoked; Whelk; Crab snow; Octopus; Croaker; Mussels;

Eggs, Beans, Nuts and Seeds

Coconut meat (dried); Seeds: cottonseed, watermelon, safflower, sesame, sunflower; Soy milk; Coconut milk; Seeds (pumpkin/squash); Egg yolk; Soybeans (dried); Soybeans (green); Egg (hard-boiled);

Instead <u>Choose</u>: Peanuts; Seeds (breadnut tree); Pigeon peas; Black-eyed peas; Other Beans; Alfalfa sprouts; Egg (duck); Chickpeas; Cashew nuts; Coconut meat (raw); Lupin; Peas (split); Egg substitute; Egg (raw);

Breads, Grains, Cereals, Pasta

Danish pastry; **Donuts**; **Muffins (blueberry)**; **Sweet rolls**; Muffins (oat bran); Croissant; Granola bars; Muffins (corn); Bread sticks; Muffins (wheat bran); Noodles: Chinese chow Mein, egg; Crackers (wheat); Melba toast; Crackers (milk); Bread (cornbread); Wheat germ; Biscuits; Rolls (hamburger/hot dog); Waffles;

Instead <u>Choose</u>: Crackers (matzo); Rolls (French); Oat bran; Spaghetti spinach; Bread (pumpernickel); Rice bran; Other Noodles; Crackers (saltines); Rice cakes; Other Bread; Cereal (granola);

Dairy Products, Fats & Oils

Hydrogenated vegetable oil; **Vegetable shortening**; **Cheese (American)**; **Margarine (less than 1 TBS of butter or margarine per day)**; **Cheese (Limburger)**; Butter (less than 1 TBS of butter or margarine per day); Oil (Ucuhuba Butter); Various Cheese; Cheese spread; Milk (chocolate); Margarine-like spreads; Non-dairy creamers; Oils: palm, cottonseed, Cocoa Butter, Babassu; Fat (chicken, turkey & duck); Lard; Various Oils; Fat (beef/lamb/pork); Cheese (Cottage); Cheese (limit to less than one serving per week for AD); Cream (whipped);

Instead <u>*Choose*</u>: *Milk (2% fat); Milk (whole); Sour cream; Oils: canola, coconut, safflower;*

Desserts, Snacks, Beverages

Cake (chocolate); **Puff pastry**; **Dessert toppings**; **Carob (candy)**; **Brownies**; **Cheesecake**; **Cookies (chocolate chip)**; **Cream puffs/Éclair**; **Candies**; **Chocolate mousse**; **After-dinner mints**; **Pie (vanilla cream)**; **Coffeecake**; **Pie (pumpkin)**; **Cake (pound)**; **Frostings**; **Various Pies**; **Ice cream (chocolate)**; **Cookies (butter)**; **Cake (shortcake)**; **Halvah (candy)**; **Sweets (4 or less servings/week) for AD**; **Cakes**; **Chewing gum**; **Cookies**; **Chocolate (sweet)**; **Jams & Preserves**; **Jellies**; **Sherbet**; **Marshmallows**; **Ice cream cones**; **Ice cream (vanilla)**; **Pudding**; **Peanut butter**; **Pancakes**; **Frozen yogurt**; **Beer**; Applesauce; Crème de menthe; Cake (angel food); Soft (carbonated) drinks; Ginger ale; Hot chocolate; Eggnog; Piña colada; Taro chips; 80+ proof distilled alc. bev.; Fruit punch; Lemonade; Whiskey; Coffee liqueur; Pie crust; Fruit leather/rolls; Tonic water; Molasses; Red Bull (drink); Sports drinks; Chocolate (dark); Potato sticks; Honey; Milk shakes; Malted drinks (nonalcoholic);

Instead <u>*Choose*</u>: *Tea (herbal); Pretzels;*

Herbs & Spices, Fast Foods, Prepared Foods

Teriyaki sauce; **Hot dog**; **Soy sauce**; **Salad dressings**; **Beef broth & stock**; **Foie gras or liver pate**; **Chicken Nuggets**; **Soup (beef barley)**; **Soup (veg/beef)**; **Miso**; **Tempeh**; **Syrup (chocolate)**; **Chicken broth**; **Tofu (fried)**; **Hamburger**; **Cheeseburger**; Breaded shrimp; Fast foods (limit to less than one serving/week); Chicken stock; Barbecue sauce; Nachos; Hush puppies; Sausage (meatless); Onion rings; Pizza; Sugar (table, powder); Tahini; Gravies (canned); Sugar (brown); Syrups; Soup (chicken noodle); Pickle (sweet); French toast; Fish stock; Potato salad; Ketchup; French fries; Mayonnaise; Sauces; Hummus; Salt (table); Natto; Hash brown potatoes; Soup (clam chowder); Taco shells; Egg rolls (veg); Poppy seed;

Instead <u>*Choose*</u>: *Dill weed; Succotash; Sage; Cottonseed meal; Balsamic vinegar; Herbs & Spices; Horseradish; Pickle; Sugar (maple); Tomato paste; Vinegar; Kimchi; Potato pancakes; Mustard; Soups: minestrone, tomato, vegetable; Sauerkraut; Corn cakes; Sauces: cheese, pepper or hot, tomato, Tabasco sauce; Capers;*

Alternative Therapies & Miscellaneous

Excess body weight (avoid low carb diets for Gout); **Deep-fried foods (limit to less than one serving/week for AD)**; **2+ alcoholic drinks/day**; **Fasting (for a specific period, don't skip meals)**; Smoking/Tobacco; Aspirin; Corn syrup (avoid drinks with added sweeteners); Smoked fish/foods; High dosages of Niacin; Prescription drugs (diuretics such as thiazide); Stress;

Key Nutrients & Herbal Meds

Brewer's Yeast; Alcohol; Fat (saturated); Omega-6 fatty acid (LA); Purine; Sugar (fructose); Sugar (refined); Trans fatty acids;

Cancer Risk (& Gout)

Cells are the building block of every organ in our body. Cells reproduce or die at varying rates depending on the organ and our age. Sometimes we have abnormal cells that reproduce or divide at a faster rate than we need. This phenomenon results in a collection of unwanted cells called a tumor. If the cells in the tumor have the ability to infiltrate other tissues and organs in our body then this tumor is considered malignant, otherwise it is considered benign. Cancer is the condition that corresponds to the malignant tumors. Cancer refers to as many as 200 different diseases but they all have the out of control cell reproduction in common.

Cancers are named after the organ where a tumor first appears. Some cancers do not form a tumor such as cancer of blood. In medical jargon, if cancer affects soft tissues and organs such as breast or lung, they are categorized as Carcinomas. If cancer affects hard tissues such as bone or muscle, they are called Sarcomas. If cancer affects our lymphatic system (i.e., part of body's circulatory system which transports things such as plasma, fats, white cells from one place to another throughout our body), it is called Lymphoma. And finally if cancer affects tissues such as blood or bone marrow, it is known as Leukemia.

There has been significant progress in cancer research and treatment of cancer over the recent decades. We understand that gene mutations are the cause of cancer development. We also know of most of the causes for gene mutations that cause cancer, i.e., the carcinogens. In short, the research has led to identification of various risk factors that increase the possibility of developing cancer. The most common of which are: family history of cancer; age (growing older); exposure to Ultraviolet (UV) radiation (from sun, tanning booths, sunlamps); certain infections; hormones (e.g., estrogen); exposure to certain chemicals (e.g., radon gas, asbestos); alcohol; tobacco; poor diet; stress; obesity and lack of physical activity. Having several risk factors does NOT mean that one will get cancer. Conversely, absence of risk factors does not mean that one will not get cancer.

The suggestions and information presented in this book are primarily focused on <u>prevention</u> of various cancer types through avoidance of the known risk factors for the specific cancer type. When known, information about food items or actions that could shrink or slow down growth of tumors is included. It is important to note that, there is no definitive cure, treatment or preventive measure that is known and certain for any specific type of cancer at this time.

Few words on phytochemicals, antioxidants, free radicals …

Phytochemicals are substances or compounds found in many plants. They are also known by other names among them antioxidants and flavonoids. While thousands of phytochemicals have been discovered, very few have been studied in detail. Some of the better known phytochemicals (antioxidants) are beta carotene, Vitamin C, folic acid and Vitamin E.

Various studies and many experts suggest that the risk of cancer can be significantly reduced by eating more fruits, vegetables, beans and whole grains that contain phytochemicals. There is some evidence that certain phytochemicals may prevent formation of tumors, or suppress cancer development. But there is no data that supports taking phytochemical supplements is as effective as consuming fruits, vegetables, beans and grains as part of a normal diet. Nor are supplements regulated by the FDA. Thus, taking phytochemicals in form of supplements is not recommended.

One group of these compounds, known as antioxidants, may protect our cells against free radicals. Free radicals are molecules produced by our body as it breaks down food or by exposure to things such as tobacco smoke or radiation. Free radicals can damage our cell's DNA and are linked to certain diseases including cancer. Antioxidants are thought to eliminate free radicals, and slow down oxidation, which is a natural process that leads to damage to the cells and tissue in our body.

Another group of these compounds is known as flavonoids. Some studies suggest that some of these compounds may protect against hormone-dependent cancers such as breast and prostate cancers. Another group of flavonoids act as antioxidants, and thus have protective and anti-cancer properties.

A third group of Phytochemicals, called Allyl Sulfides, may help our body get rid of harmful chemicals and strengthen our immune system.

Many of the dietary recommendations that you find in this book are based on the various known phytochemical content and their effect on various types of cancer.

General Considerations for Defeating Cancer

Despite all the advances made in cancer research over the last several decades, per 2012 estimates from American Cancer Society (ACS), one third of Americans diagnosed with cancer die within the first five years. Considering there is over 1.6 million new cases of cancer per annum (2012 ACS estimate), this translates to an unacceptably high number of fatalities, and is a clear indication of inadequacy of existing capabilities to prevent and treat this terrible disease. In a nutshell, the prevailing cancer treatment is based on either surgery to remove affected tissue and organs, or destruction of our body cells through chemotherapy and radiation with the hope that the cancer cells will also get killed in the process. There are newer treatment paradigms emerging (e.g., cancer vaccines and adoptive immunotherapy which are the personalized medicine approaches to cancer treatment) but they are just that, too new and emerging. There has been very limited curative treatments to-date, and only in clinical trials.

Much too often patients die from the cancer treatment and not the cancer. Much too often patients refuse treatment due to unacceptable side effects, unacceptable risk-reward ratio, or because they are too weak to receive further treatment.

On the other hand, per ACS estimate, environmental factors (i.e., factors that we can control) account for 75-80% of cancer cases and deaths in the US. We need to recognize these factors and take appropriate action to avoid them and reduce our risk of getting cancer.

A common criticism of the conventional approach to cancer is that diet, free-radicals, toxins and other environmental factors are neglected. Medical community and the Pharmaceutical industry are focused on eliminating cancer cells, not cancer-causing factors. As a result, for the foreseeable future, we must take it upon ourselves to take actions to reduce our risk of getting cancer. And until there is further progress in conventional approach to cancer treatment, cancer patients and the health care community must actively seek and further explore various alternative and complementary medicine (ACM) and therapies available to them. A number of western European countries and China have successfully integrated ACM into the conventional approach to prevention and treatment of cancer.

While the focus of this book is on nutrition, we will also mention various herbal remedies and complementary therapies that are available to you. It is beyond the scope of this book, to discuss all these options in detail. But we highly encourage you to learn about these ACMs and discuss them with your natural health care provider.

To combat cancer we must recognize the main factors identified as culprits and develop an action plan to deal with each. The factors most often mentioned include: nutritional deficiencies, environmental toxins, stress, smoking, free radicals, and excess weight. Recent studies have also found a link between inflammation (our immune system natural reaction to injuries, allergies, germs and the like) and cancer.

For dealing with environmental toxins and free radicals attributed to pollution, chemicals and smoking, there are a number of detoxification programs, multi-day fasts or cleansing diets that are explicitly designed to address this critical need. There are also a number of nutrients and foods that are considered helpful in detoxification of our body, and are mentioned separately in this book.

As for the remaining factors, the guidelines provided in this book are designed to augment a well-balanced diet with antioxidants or cancer fighting foods, boost your immune system, and minimize or eliminate the damage from free radicals that are created through your food intake. Separate guidelines are also provided for dealing with obesity and stress.

One nutrition-centric approach that has been controversial but worthy of further investigation is a diet that is focused on increasing the alkalinity (or reducing the acidity) of our body tissue. There are a number of studies that suggest that the cancer cells are less likely to survive an alkaline tissue environment. A separate chapter on alkaline diet is included in this book.

There are a number of factors that are considered by some as culprits in causing cancer. While there are some books and reports published on these factors, there remains some skepticism and controversy about accuracy of such claims. But for the sake of completeness, we are including this list of suspects for your information: prescription and non-prescription drugs (due to chemical toxins), micro-waved foods, fast foods, various soda (since they can block absorption of certain nutrients), high fructose syrups, non-stick cookware, farmed fish and non-organic meat and poultry (due to growth hormones, antibiotics and chemicals fed to these animals), pork, shellfish, skin care lotions including sun-block creams, deodorants, air fresheners, all man-made and processed foods, swimming pools & steam rooms (due to chlorine), and fluorescent lighting.

In closing, remember that it is your body and it is your life. Your best ally is a strong immune system. Take actions to boost it. Remain skeptical of anyone who promises a miracle cure. And remain just as skeptical of anyone who dismisses other approaches too quickly in favor of their own. No single organization, clinic, or expert has the monopoly on the truth when it comes to cancer. And considering that cancer represents a several hundred billion dollars per year business in the US, far too many experts and organizations have a conflict of interest in their position on how to deal with cancer.

Choose these for Gout & Cancer Risk

Top 5 items to consume:

> **Organic Fruits, Berries & Juices; Pure water; Tofu; Red Cabbage & Other Leafy Vegetables; Peppers;**

Food items & actions that could improve your health or reduce your risk (within a food group, most helpful items are listed first):

Meat, Fish & Poultry

Sturgeon; Conch; Pompano fish; Spot;

Eggs, Beans, Nuts and Seeds

Peas (sugar/snap); Beans: yardlong, navy, hyacinth; Peas (green); Seeds (flaxseed; take ground seeds with water); Walnuts; Beans (fava); Chickpeas; Other Beans; Pigeon peas; Lentils; Seeds (breadnut tree); Soybeans (green); Black-eyed peas; Seeds (chia); Soy milk; Peas (split); Alfalfa sprouts;

Fruits & Juices (Five servings of fruits & vegetables daily)

Avoid non-organic. Avoid sugared juices or from concentrate; Wash fruits & vegetables well and peel their skin; Cranberries; Cranberry juice; Currants (raw); Orange juice; Rhubarb; Oranges; Various Berries; Guava; Lemon; Persimmons; Pomegranate; Acerola; Cherries (especially tart and including juice); Grapefruit; Kumquats; Pumelo (Shaddock); Grapefruit juice; Rowal; Papaya; Jujube (fruit); Litchi; Longans; Peaches; Abiyuch; Plum; Nectarine; Kiwi fruit; Tamarind; Mango; Litchi (dried); Olives; Plantains; Pineapple; Lime; Currants (dried); Breadfruit; Pitanga; Natal Plum (Carissa); Tangerines; Watermelon; Starfruit; Cantaloupe; Apples; Avocado; Pineapple juice; Peaches (dried); Durian; Passion fruit; Pears (dried); Apples (dried); Apricots; Apricots (dried); Figs; Dried fruits; Apple juice; Grapes; Quince; Grape juice; Banana; Pomegranate juice; Honeydew melon; Pears; Prune juice; Dates; Raisins;

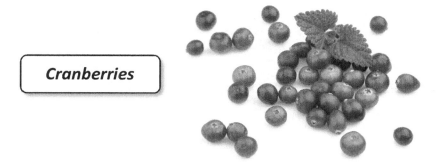

Cranberries

Vegetables (Five servings of fruits & vegetables daily)

Avoid non-organic. Wash fruits & vegetables well and peel their skin; Peppers (hot chili, red); Cabbage (red); Tomato juice; Balsam pear leafy tips; Garden cress; Lambsquarters; Mustard spinach; Peppers; Pokeberry shoots; Sesbania Flower; Taro (Tahitian); Taro leaves; Vine spinach (Basella); Cabbage (green); Amaranth leaves; Watercress; Winged beans leaves; Yam; Cabbage (savoy); Borage; Cowpeas leafy tips; Dandelion Greens; Tomatoes; Bell peppers (red); Kohlrabi; Beet greens; Pumpkin flowers; Squash (Butternut); Sweet potatoes; Swiss chard; Squash (Acorn); Chicory greens; Okra; Purslane; Turnip greens; Bell peppers (green); Arugula; Broccoli; Celtuce; Green onions (scallions); Bok choy; Parsnips; Chrysanthemum (Garland); Chrysanthemum Leaves; Endive; Epazote; Grape leaves; Various Lettuce; Squash (Hubbard); Sweet potatoes leaves; Tomatoes (sun-dried); Potatoes w/skin; Brussels sprouts; Broccoli (Chinese); Radishes; Lotus root; Zucchini; Arrowroot; Mushrooms (Chanterelle); Mustard greens; Taro; Kale; Garlic (use raw or crushed but not heated immediately); Nopal; Cucumber with peel; Cloud ear fungus; Onions (2-5 oz. of fresh onions daily, or 1 tsp juice 3-4 times a day); Collards; Fennel (Bulb); Pumpkin; Kelp; Rutabaga; Turnips; Arrowhead; Shallots; Balsam pear; Cauliflower; Artichoke; Potato; Green beans; Squash (Spaghetti); Wasabi root; Mushrooms (Morel); Eggplant; Celery; Spinach; Other Mushrooms; Hearts of palm; Other vegetables;

Breads, Grains, Cereals, Pasta

Buckwheat; Quinoa; Amaranth; Triticale; Rye grain; English muffins (whole-wheat); Rice (wild); Cereal (shredded wheat); Tortillas (corn); Sorghum grain; Corn bran; Spaghetti (whole-wheat); Cereals; Oatmeal (cereal); Barley; Oats; Rice (brown); Bulgur; Bread (whole-wheat); Bread (Italian); Millet; Bread (French/Sourdough); Durum wheat; Spelt; Rolls (whole-wheat dinner); Bread (pumpernickel); Bread (oat bran); Cereal (cream of wheat); Corn; Pasta;

Dairy Products, Fats & Oils

Yogurt; Fish oil (cod liver); Whey (sweet); Cheese (Cottage); Milk (1% fat); Cream; Milk (skim); Buttermilk; Cheese (Gjetost); Sour cream; Cheese (Ricotta); choose low-fat dairy products;

Desserts, Snacks, Beverages

Water (clean water, not tap water); Popcorn (air popped); Coffee (decaf, lowers risk of gout among men); Wine (red); Tea (green, do not brew or drink boiling hot); Coffee; Tea (plain); Popcorn (oil popped); Wine (white);

Herbs & Spices, Fast Foods, Prepared Foods

Parsley; Cornmeal (whole-grain); Tofu; Thyme (fresh); Egg rolls (veg); Coriander/Cilantro; Soup (minestrone); Corn salad; Soup (vegetable); Tomato paste; Mints; Dill weed; Sauerkraut; Kimchi; Spearmint (fresh); Peppermint; Cayenne (red) pepper; Basil (fresh); Mace; Nutmeg; Rosemary (fresh); Turmeric; Soup (tomato); French fries; Succotash; Pepper (black); Potato pancakes; Balsamic vinegar; Natto; Vinegar; Sage; Sugar (maple);

Alternative Therapies & Miscellaneous

Consult your doctor (ask for screening tests); Exercise (Cardiovascular, weight training, jogging, walking, or cycling); Fluids, Juices & Water; Fresh (uncooked) fruits/veg's; Alkaline diet; Anti-inflammation diet; Organic cold-pressed oils; Organically grown foods (If non-organic, wash fruits/vegs well and peel off their skin); Wild fish and free range animals (Avoid animals raised on antibiotics or grains);

Key Nutrients & Herbal Meds

Goji berry; Beta Carotene (do not take in supplement form); Bugleweed; Celery seed; Fiber; Flavonoids; Foxglove; Psyllium; Starch/complex carbohydrates; Vitamin C;

Do not choose these for Gout & Cancer Risk

Top 5 items to avoid:

> Processed & Cured Meats; Chocolate; Pork/Beef;
> Sweets; Smoked Salmon;

Avoid or consume much less of the following (within a food group, most harmful items are listed first):

Meat, Fish & Poultry

Bacon; Cured Meats; Beef jerky sticks; Beef tongue; Salami; Bologna; Chorizo; Corned beef; Frankfurters; Luncheon meats; Pastrami; Pepperoni; Pork cured/ham; Sausages; Pork ribs; Beef (ground); Lamb ribs; Turkey skins; Lamb tongue; Pork spare ribs; Beef chuck/brisket; Salmon (smoked, Lox); Pork skins; Pork; Organ meats; Chicken skin; Beef ribs; Tuna (canned); Lamb; Veal; White fish (smoked); Game meats; Goose; Beef; Liver; Rabbit meat; Venison; Quail; Bison/buffalo meat; Scallops; Meat (limit consumption of red meat; choose organic); Goat meat; Chicken dark meat; Shark; Boar meat; Pheasant; Tuna (yellowfin); Frog legs; Squab (pigeon); Chicken wings; Perch; Croaker; Carp; Sardines; Pheasant breast; Mackerel; Quail breast; Cod; Duck (no skin); Lobster; Cisco (smoked); Orange roughy; Fish roe; Halibut; Anchovy; Grouper; Guinea hen; Caviar; Chicken breast (no skin); Shrimp; Mackerel (king); Northern pike; Turkey dark meat; Turkey breast; Monkfish; Tilefish; Dolphinfish (Mahi-Mahi); Haddock; Sablefish; Flatfish (flounder & sole); Squid (Calamari); Seatrout; Walleye; Bluefish; Herring; Tuna (blue fin); Abalone; Various Bass; Rockfish; Sheepshead; Milkfish; Marlin; Swordfish; Whelk; Clams; Cuttlefish; Mussels; Lobster (spiny); Trout; Butterfish; Pumpkinseed sunfish; Crab (snow); Burbot; Cisco; Snapper; Turbot; Yellowtail; Crab (Alaskan King); Scup; Drum; Octopus; Shad; Snail; Cusk; Ling;

Instead _Choose_: Smelt; Whiting; Wolffish; Crab (Dungeness); Oysters; Catfish; Lingcod; Surimi; Mullet; Tilapia; Eel; White fish; Salmon (pink); Pollock; Pout; Crab (Blue); Crayfish; Bass (freshwater); Sucker;

Eggs, Beans, Nuts and Seeds

Cashew nuts; Pili nuts; Butternuts; Seeds (pumpkin/squash); Hickory nuts; Peanuts; Pine nuts; Walnuts (black); Seeds: watermelon, cottonseed, sesame; Coconut meat (dried); Soybeans (dried); Pistachio nuts; Brazil nuts; Coconut meat (raw); Pecans; Seeds (safflower); Coconut milk; Beechnuts; Macadamia nuts; Seeds (sunflower); Cornnuts; Acorns;

Instead _Choose_: Egg substitute; Egg (duck); Lupin; Ginkgo nuts; Egg white; Breadfruit seeds; Chestnuts; Egg (raw); Egg (hard-boiled); Hazelnuts or Filberts; Almonds; Egg yolk;

Breads, Grains, Cereals, Pasta

Danish pastry; **Sweet rolls**; **Donuts**; **Muffins (blueberry)**; **Wheat germ**; **Granola bars**; Muffins (oat bran); Croissant; Muffins (wheat bran); Various Crackers; Cereal (granola); Wheat bran; Wheat; Bread sticks; Rolls (hamburger/hot dog); Muffins (corn); Semolina; Biscuits; Whole-wheat; Noodles (Chinese chow Mein); Rice (white); Melba toast; Noodles (egg); Couscous; Bagels; Rice bran;

Instead <u>*Choose*</u>: *Toasted bread; Waffles; Bread (wheat germ); Spaghetti (spinach); Spaghetti; Rice cakes (Brown rice); Oat bran; English muffins; Bread (cornbread); Bread (banana); Bread (white); Crackers (whole-wheat); Noodles (Japanese); Noodles (rice);*

Dairy Products, Fats & Oils

Vegetable shortening; **Milk (chocolate)**; **Hydrogenated vegetable oil**; **Cheese (American)**; **Non-dairy creamers**; Butter (salted); Oil: wheat germ, Ucuhuba Butter; Margarine; Butter (unsalted); Fat (duck, chicken, turkey); Lard; Oil (coconut); Cheese (Romano); Various Oils; Fat (beef/lamb/pork); Cheese spread; Cheese (Parmesan); Cheese (Blue); Various Cheese; Margarine-like spreads; Cream (whipped); Oils: almonds, safflower;

Instead <u>*Choose*</u>: *Various Fish oil; Milk (2% fat); Milk (whole); Cheese (Swiss); Oil (flaxseed); Oil (hazelnut);*

Desserts, Snacks, Beverages

Cake (chocolate); **Cookies (chocolate chip)**; **Cream puffs/Éclair**; **Puff pastry**; **Candies (peanut bar)**; **Brownies**; **Peanut butter**; **Dessert toppings**; **Halvah (candy)**; **Coffee liqueur**; **Coffeecake**; **Cheesecake**; **Pudding**; **Cookies (butter)**; **Cakes**; **Chocolate mousse**; **Soft (carbonated) drinks**; **Pie (fried, fruit)**; **Crème de menthe**; **Candies**; **Ice cream (chocolate)**; **Various Pies**; **Red Bull (drink)**; **After-dinner mints**; **Cookies**; **Applesauce**; **Chocolate (sweet)**; **Hot chocolate**; **Frostings**; **Carob (candy)**; **Ice cream cones**; **Ginger ale**; **Chewing gum**; **Molasses**; **Fruit leather/rolls**; **Marshmallows**; **Eggnog**; **Lemonade**; **80+ proof distilled alc. bev.**; Fruit punch; Sherbet; Candies (hard); Piña colada; Jams & Preserves; Jellies; Tonic water; Ice cream (vanilla); Beer; Pancakes; Chocolate (dark); Honey; Taro chips; Frozen yogurt; Whiskey; Sports drinks; Pie crust; Pie (pumpkin); Milk shakes; Potato sticks; Tortilla chips; Pretzels;

Instead <u>*choose*</u>: *Tea (herbal); Potato chips; Malted drinks (nonalcoholic);*

Herbs & Spices, Fast Foods, Prepared Foods

Hot dog; **Barbecue sauce**; **Sugar (table, powder)**; **Salad dressings**; **Chicken Nuggets**; **Beef broth & Stock**; **Foie gras or liver pate**; **Syrup (chocolate)**; **Soup (beef barley)**; **Teriyaki sauce**; **Sausage (meatless)**; **Syrups**; **Sauce (Hoisin)**; **Ketchup**; **Sugar (brown)**; **Pickle (sweet)**; **Cheeseburger**; Breaded shrimp; Tahini; Nachos; **Hamburger**; Soy sauce; Hush puppies; Onion rings; Pizza; Sauces; Gravies (canned); Chicken broth & Stock; Sauce (fish); Tabasco sauce; Syrup (maple); Fish stock; Tofu (fried); Soup (chicken noodle); Sauce (pepper or hot); Soup (clam chowder); French toast; Sauce (tomato); Mayonnaise; Hummus; Croutons; Salt (table); Potato salad; Miso; Corn cakes; Taco shells; Soup (veg/beef); Macaroni; Hash brown potatoes; Pickle relish; Cottonseed meal;

Instead <u>*Choose*</u>*: Chervil; Ginger; Horseradish; Marjoram; Tarragon; Cole slaw;*

Tempeh; Cardamom; Chives; Cinnamon; Cloves; Oregano; Saffron; Fennel seeds; Pickle (cucumber); Mustard seed; Poppy seed; Capers; Falafel; Mustard; Cocoa;

Alternative Therapies & Miscellaneous

2+ alcoholic drinks/day; **Excess body weight (avoid low carb diets)**; **Smoked Fish/Food**; **Smoking/Tobacco**; **Corn syrup**; **Fasting (for a specific period; don't skip meals)**; **Deep fried foods**; **Pesticide-loaded crops (avoid non-organic foods. if not possible, wash fruits/vegs well and peel off their skin)**; **Processed or Refined foods**; Prescription drugs (diuretics such as thiazide); Air pollutants; Food additives Nitrates/Nitrites; Harsh chemicals & fumes; High dosages of Niacin; Non-organic foods; Radiation (from X-rays, TV, microwave, computer, cell phones); Stress;

Key Nutrients & Herbal Meds

Brewer's Yeast; **Sugar (fructose)**; **Sugar (refined)**; **Trans fatty acids**; Alcohol; Betel Nut; Mercury (avoid heavy metal loaded fish); Purine; Fat (saturated); Caffeine;

Stress (& Gout)

Everyone experiences some sort of stress almost every day. Stress is our brain's response to a demand. Not everyone reacts to the same events or demands the same way. What may be stressful to one person may not be to another. It is stress that drives us to act, and in some cases such as survival situations, perform beyond our normal abilities. However, long term or chronic stress can lead to a variety of problems including illnesses such as high blood pressure, depression and cancer.

Chronic stress can be caused by a number of factors, among them: bad childhood experiences (whose pain and impact you have never been able to escape), poverty and helplessness, an unhappy marriage, never-ending tension and violence all around you, a wrong job or career, and a dysfunctional family.

Chronic stress challenges our mind and body over a long time, and thus may require an on-going treatment over an extended period of time.

Choose these for Gout & Stress

Top 5 items to consume:

>Cereals; Fruits and Juices; Red Cabbage & Other Leafy Vegetables; Hot Peppers; Tofu; & Exercise;

Food items and actions that could improve your health (within a food group, most helpful items are listed first):

Meat, Fish & Poultry

Surimi; Various Bass; Bluefish; Butterfish; Catfish; Cisco; Cusk; Drum; Lingcod; Mackerel (king); Marlin; Milkfish; Mullet; Pollock; Pumpkinseed sunfish; Rockfish; Scup; Seatrout; Shad; Sheepshead; Smelt; Snapper; Spot; Sturgeon; Sucker; Swordfish; Tilapia; Tilefish; Whiting; Wolffish; Burbot; Conch; Octopus; Whelk; Ling; Dolphinfish (Mahi-Mahi); Grouper; Turbot; Pompano fish; Sablefish; Snail; Cuttlefish; Yellowtail; Shark; Monkfish; Pout; Clams; Veal thymus; Eel; Beef spleen; Crab (Dungeness); Lobster (spiny); Turkey liver; Flatfish (flounder & sole); White fish; Oysters; Haddock; Beef round steak; Crab (Alaskan King); Crab (Blue); Beaver meat; Beef filet mignon; Orange roughy; Caribou meat; Veal spleen; Crab (snow); Beef tenderloin/T-bone/porterhouse; Carp; Halibut; Northern pike; Perch; Salmon (pink); Trout; Tuna (blue fin); Tuna (yellowfin); Walleye; Croaker; Veal shank; Crayfish; Pork loin/sirloin; Chicken breast (no skin); Chicken liver; Beef rib eye; Rabbit meat; Beef top sirloin; Cod;

Eggs, Beans, Nuts and Seeds

Peas: sugar/snap, green; Egg (duck); Egg yolk; Seeds (chia); Egg (hard-boiled); Seeds (breadnut tree); Egg (raw); Seeds (flaxseed); Beans (yardlong); Egg white; Beans (hyacinth); Seeds (safflower);

Fruits & Juices

Orange juice; Currants (raw); Acerola; Guava; Jujube (fruit); Lemon; Longans; Persimmons; Pumelo (Shaddock); Kumquats; Grapefruit juice; Oranges; Litchi; Strawberries; Abiyuch; Papaya; Litchi (dried); Pineapple; Cherries especially tart including juice); Tamarind; Natal Plum (Carissa); Mulberries; Kiwi fruit; Pomegranate; Breadfruit; Raspberries; Lime; Starfruit; Avocado; Rowal; Nectarine; Grapefruit; Banana; Currants (dried); Berries; Peaches; Cantaloupe; Cranberry juice; Plantains; Apple juice; Plum; Prune juice; Durian; Passion fruit; Olives; Dried fruits; Mango; Pitanga; Pineapple juice; Cranberries; Watermelon; Apples; Pomegranate juice; Raisins; Tangerines; Grape juice; Grapes; Dates; Rhubarb; Pears; Honeydew melon; Quince; Figs; Apricots; **Avoid sugared and made from concentrate juices;**

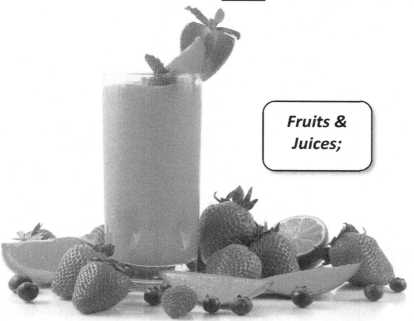

Fruits & Juices;

Vegetables

Peppers (hot chili, red); Cabbage (red); Balsam pear; Balsam pear leafy tips; Garden cress; Lambsquarters; Mustard spinach; Peppers; Pokeberry shoots; Sesbania Flower; Taro (Tahitian); Taro leaves; Vine spinach (Basella); Amaranth leaves; Winged beans leaves; Bell peppers (red); Kohlrabi; Cowpeas leafy tips; Yam; Broccoli; Borage; Bok choy; Cabbage (green); Grape leaves; Watercress; Brussels sprouts; Bell peppers (green); Cabbage (savoy); Epazote; Garlic; Turnip greens; Mustard greens; Dandelion Greens; Pumpkin flowers; Lotus root; Cauliflower; Squash (Acorn); Broccoli (Chinese); Purslane; Potatoes w/skin; Kale; Arrowhead; Shallots; Arugula; Chicory greens; Kelp; Sweet potatoes leaves; Arrowroot; Beet greens; Tomato juice; Chrysanthemum (Garland); Chrysanthemum Leaves; Mushrooms (Chanterelle); Fiddlehead ferns; Green onions (scallions); Taro; Onions; Tomatoes (sun-dried); Nopal; Celtuce; Swiss chard; Squash (Butternut); Cucumber with peel; Cloud ear fungus; Collards; Okra; Radishes; Potato; Mushrooms (Morel); Fennel (Bulb); Sweet potatoes; Artichoke (Jerusalem); Hearts of palm; Carrots; Various Lettuce; Rutabaga; Wasabi root; Parsnips; Tomatoes; Mushrooms; Turnips; Squash (Hubbard); Spinach; Celery; Zucchini; Artichoke; Squash (Spaghetti);

Breads, Grains, Cereals, Pasta

Cereals: rice crisps, corn flakes, shredded wheat, raisin bran; English muffins (whole-wheat); Other Cereals; Quinoa; Rice bran; Tortillas (corn); Rice (wild); Triticale; Bread (whole-wheat); Oatmeal (cereal); Spelt; English muffins; Bagels; Toasted bread; Spaghetti (whole-wheat); Rye grain; Rice cakes (Brown rice); Bulgur; Waffles; Wheat bran; Bread (French/Sourdough); Rolls (whole-wheat dinner); Millet; Bread (Italian); Spaghetti; Buckwheat; Bread (cornbread); Sorghum grain; Rice (white); Bread (white); Bread (wheat germ); Biscuits; Corn bran; Amaranth; Rice (brown); Bread (pumpernickel); Bread (oat bran); Durum wheat; Whole-wheat; Semolina; Muffins (oat bran); Oats;

Dairy Products, Fats & Oils

Milk (skim); Milk (1% fat); Cheese (Swiss); Cheese (Gruyere); Yogurt; Various Cheese; Cream; Milk (2% fat); Fish oil (cod liver); Buttermilk; Whey (sweet); Milk (whole); Sour cream; Cheese (Camembert); Cheese spread; Fish oil (salmon); Fish oil (sardine);

Desserts, Snacks, Beverages

Popcorn (air popped); **Water**; **Potato chips**; Coffee (decaf, lowers risk of Gout for men); Tortilla chips; Potato sticks; Popcorn (oil popped); Coffee; Pretzels; Tea (green, decaf in particular); Candies (sesame crunch); Fruit leather/rolls;

Herbs & Spices, Fast Foods, Prepared Foods

Cornmeal (whole-grain); **Tofu**; **Potato pancakes**; **Corn salad**; Cottonseed meal; Taco shells; Thyme (fresh); Ginger; Parsley; Egg rolls (veg); Natto; Kimchi; Hash brown potatoes; Corn cakes; Succotash; Dill weed; Sauerkraut; Cole slaw; French fries; Nachos;

Alternative Therapies & Miscellaneous

Consult your doctor (determine if you suffer from adrenal fatigue); **Exercise (Including Cardiovascular, Weight Training, Walking, Jogging, or Cycling)**; **Fluids/Juices/Water;** Fresh (uncooked) fruits/veg's; Laugh, laughter; Meditation; Organically grown foods; Sleep 6-8 hours regularly; Take a vacation!; Yoga;

Key Nutrients & Herbal Meds

Vitamin C; **Starch/complex carbohydrates**; Ashwaganda (root & leaf); Calcium; Celery seed; Ginseng (Asian); Ginseng (Siberian); Licorice root; Magnesium; Vitamin B-6 (Pyridoxine); Vitamin D;

Do not choose these for Gout & Stress

Top 5 items to avoid:

Chocolate; Beer; Sweets; Luncheon (processed) Meats; Teriyaki & Soy Sauces; & 2+ Alcoholic drinks/day;

Avoid or consume much less of the following (within a food group, most harmful items are listed first):

Meat, Fish & Poultry

Sausages; **Luncheon meats**; **Frankfurters**; **Pastrami**; **Pepperoni**; **Salami**; **Chicken skin**; **Chorizo**; **Beef jerky sticks**; **Corned beef**; **Cured Meats**; **Pork skins**; **Bologna**; **Pork breakfast strips**; **Bacon**; Pork cured/ham; Goose; Beef tongue; Turkey skins; Beef (cured dried); Organ meats; Duck (no skin); Quail; Pork ribs; Chicken dark meat; Lamb ribs; Pork; Scallops; Quail breast; Squab (pigeon); Liver; Guinea hen; Chicken wings; Frog legs; Beef chuck/brisket; Fish roe; Pheasant; Tuna (canned); Venison; Caviar; Pheasant breast; Turkey breast; Lamb leg; Salmon (smoked, Lox);

Instead **choose**: Mussels; Cisco (smoked); White fish (smoked); Beef shank; Bison/buffalo meat; Goat meat; Boar meat; Anchovy; Herring; Mackerel; Sardines; Shrimp; Abalone; Veal loin; Lamb shoulder; Turkey dark meat; Lamb (ground); Lamb loin; Veal shoulder; Squid (Calamari); Pork back ribs; Lobster; Beef (ground);

Eggs, Beans, Nuts and Seeds

Peanuts; **Pili nuts**; Hickory nuts; Butternuts; Beechnuts; Beans (black); Pecans; Pine nuts; Acorns; Breadfruit seeds; Cornnuts; Cashew nuts; Coconut meat (dried); Soybeans (green); Chestnuts; Coconut meat (raw); Ginkgo nuts; Macadamia nuts; Soybeans (dried); Beans: adzuki, lima; Pistachio nuts; Walnuts (black); Beans (navy); Walnuts; Beans (kidney); Peas (split); Beans (baked); Lupin; Coconut milk; Chickpeas; Alfalfa sprouts; Soy milk; Brazil nuts; Pigeon peas; Beans (Great Northern); Lentils; Beans: pinto, mung;

Instead **Choose**: Beans (fava); Seeds (cottonseed); Beans (winged); Seeds (sunflower); Almonds; Egg substitute; Seeds (watermelon); Beans (yellow); Seeds (pumpkin/squash); Hazelnuts or Filberts; Seeds (sesame); Beans (moth beans); Black-eyed peas;

Vegetables

Leeks; Asparagus; Green beans; Endive

Instead **Choose**: Eggplant; Pumpkin; Beets;

Breads, Grains, Cereals, Pasta

Danish pastry; **Sweet rolls**; **Donuts**; **Muffins (blueberry)**; Croissant; Crackers (wheat); Granola bars; Crackers (milk); Noodles (egg); Wheat germ; Melba toast; Bread sticks; Other Crackers; Corn; Barley; Noodles (Chinese chow Mein); Cereal (granola); Muffins (corn); Rolls (Kaiser); Noodles (rice); Wheat;

Instead **choose**: Spaghetti (spinach); Muffins (wheat bran); Pasta; Oat bran; Bread (banana); Noodles (Japanese); Cereal (cream of wheat); Crackers (whole-wheat); Couscous; Croutons;

Dairy Products, Fats & Oils

Milk (chocolate); **Hydrogenated vegetable oil**; **Margarine**; **Non-dairy creamers**; Vegetable shortening; Oils: coconut, Ucuhuba Butter; Margarine-like spreads; Fat (duck, chicken, turkey); Lard; Oils: Cocoa Butter, Cupu Assu, tea seed; Other Oils; Fat (beef/lamb/pork); Butter; Oil (sunflower); Oil (olive); Oil (canola);

*Instead **choose**: Cheese (Limburger); Fish oils; Oils: flaxseed, hazelnut, safflower, almonds; Cheese: Brie, Ricotta, Goat, Cream; Cream (whipped); Milk shakes;*

Desserts, Snacks, Beverages

Cake (chocolate); **Puff pastry**; **Chocolate (dark)**; **Cookies (chocolate chip)**; **Ice cream (chocolate)**; **Brownies**; **Chocolate mousse**; **Cream puffs/Éclair**; **Coffee liqueur**; **Cheesecake**; **Chocolate (sweet)**; **Coffeecake**; **Candies (peanut brittle)**; **Hot chocolate**; **Pudding**; **Crème de menthe**; **Dessert toppings**; **Cakes**; **Pie (fried, fruit)**; **Beer**; **After-dinner mints**; **Cookies**; **Applesauce**; **Frostings**; **Peanut butter**; **Pie (vanilla cream)**; **80+ proof distilled alc. bev.**; **Whiskey**; **Fruit punch**; **Soft (carbonated) drinks**; **Piña colada**; **Chewing gum**; **Pie (coconut cream)**; **Ginger ale**; Cookies (animal crackers); Other Pies; Ice cream cones; Candies; Lemonade; Jams & Preserves; Sherbet; Marshmallows; Carob (candy); Jellies; Eggnog; Ice cream (vanilla); Tonic water; Sports drinks; Honey; Halvah (candy); Frozen yogurt; Red Bull (drink); Tea (plain); Malted drinks (nonalcoholic); Wine (red); Wine (white); Pie crust; Taro chips;

*Instead **choose**: Molasses; Tea (herbal); Pancakes; Milk shakes;*

Herbs & Spices, Fast Foods, Prepared Foods

Teriyaki sauce; **Soy sauce**; **Salad dressings**; **Hot dog**; **Syrup (chocolate)**; **Barbecue sauce**; **Miso**; **Sugar (table, powder)**; **Foie gras or liver pate**; **Chicken Nuggets**; Sugar (brown); Syrup (table blends); Tofu (fried); Ketchup; Tahini; Soup (beef barley); Sauce (Hoisin); Beef broth & stock; Chicken broth & stock; Gravies (canned); Pickle (sweet); Syrup (maple); Tempeh; Cocoa; Potato salad; Fish stock; Sauces; Mayonnaise; Soups: chicken noodle, veg/beef, vegetable, minestrone; Syrup (malt); Poppy seed; Tomato paste; Turmeric; Sausage (meatless); French toast; Onion rings; Breaded shrimp; Pizza; Soup (tomato); Salt (table); Cloves;

*Instead **choose**: Falafel; Mints; Hush puppies; Falafel; Hush puppies; Rosemary & Sage; Pickle; Cheeseburger; Macaroni; Syrup (Sorghum); Balsamic vinegar; Herbs & Spices; Horseradish; Sugar (maple); Vinegar; Hummus; Mustard; Hamburger; Capers; Soup (clam chowder);*

Alternative Therapies & Miscellaneous

2+ alcoholic drinks/day; **Excess body weight**; **Fasting (for a specific period; do not skip meals)**; Deep-fried foods; Prescription drugs (diuretics such as thiazide); Corn syrup; Aspirin; Smoked fish/foods; High dosages of Niacin; Smoking/Tobacco;

Key Nutrients & Herbal Meds

Brewer's Yeast; Alcohol; Sugar (refined); Purine; Sugar (fructose); Oxalate; Caffeine; Fat (saturated);

Vitamin D Deficiency (& Gout)

Vitamin D Deficiency is a common problem for many people especially the older people. Vitamin D is a critical nutrient for your body in particular for stronger bones, muscle movements, nerve function and immune system well-being.

You will develop this deficiency if you don't absorb enough Vitamin D from your diet, you don't get enough exposure to the sun (especially during the winter months), your skin cannot convert the sun exposure to Vitamin D (as in elderly and darker skin), or you are obese. You can also develop this deficiency if your body cannot properly process fats due to Celiac or Crohn's disease, since fats are required for Vitamin D absorption into your blood. Health issues with kidney and liver can also result in this deficiency because they can prevent your body to process Vitamin D.

Adults, ages 19 to 70, require 600 IU (International Units) of Vitamin D per day. Adults, ages 71 and above, require 800 IU per day.

Meeting your Vitamin D needs entirely through sun exposure or tanning is not recommended due to the risk of skin cancer. Too much Vitamin D in your blood (almost always caused by supplements) can also be harmful.

Choose these for Gout & Vitamin D Deficiency

Top 5 items to consume:

> Corn Flakes/Cereals; Water & Fruit Juice; Cherries & Currants; Peppers, Mushrooms & Yam; Cod Liver Fish Oil; ... and Exposure to Sun

Food items and actions that could improve your health (within a food group, most helpful items are listed first):

Meat, Fish & Poultry

Catfish; Marlin; Snapper; Sturgeon; Swordfish; Pompano fish; Eel; White fish; Carp; Salmon (pink); Trout; Bass (seabass); Shad;

Eggs, Beans, Nuts and Seeds

Egg yolk; Soy milk; There are no other items in this food group that can help your conditions. See the next section for neutral items.

Fruits & Juices

Cherries (especially tart, including juice); Cranberry juice; Cranberries; Orange juice; Currants (raw); Rhubarb; Berries; Oranges; Grapefruit juice; Acerola; Guava; Jujube (fruit); Lemon; Litchi; Longans; Persimmons; Pumelo (Shaddock); Pomegranate; Avocado; Grapefruit; Kumquats; Litchi (dried); Pineapple juice; Nectarine; Pineapple; Rowal; Natal Plum (Carissa); Peaches; Currants (dried); Abiyuch; Kiwi fruit; Papaya; Plum; Breadfruit; Lime; Starfruit; Olives; Pears (dried); Tamarind; Apples; Dried fruits; Pitanga; Apple juice; Tangerines; Mango; Durian; Plantains; Grape juice; Figs; Watermelon; Pomegranate juice; Cantaloupe; Honeydew melon; Quince; Banana; Grapes; Prune juice; Dates; Pears; **Avoid sugared fruit juices or from concentrate;**

Vegetables

Peppers (hot chili, red); Mushrooms (Chanterelle); Yam; Cabbage (red); Tomato juice; Balsam pear; Balsam pear leafy tips; Garden cress; Lambsquarters; Mustard spinach; Peppers; Pokeberry shoots; Potatoes w/skin; Sesbania Flower; Taro (Tahitian); Taro leaves; Vine spinach (Basella); Cabbage (green); Amaranth leaves; Squash (Acorn); Watercress; Winged beans leaves; Mushrooms (Morel); Cabbage (savoy); Borage; Cowpeas leafy tips; Dandelion Greens; Tomatoes; Celery; Bell peppers (red); Kohlrabi; Beet greens; Parsnips; Pumpkin flowers; Squash (Butternut); Sweet potatoes; Swiss chard; Chicory greens; Lotus root; Okra; Purslane; Turnip greens; Onions; Bell peppers (green); Arugula; Broccoli; Celtuce; Fiddlehead ferns; Green onions (scallions); Bok choy; Potato; Arrowhead; Arrowroot; Artichoke (Jerusalem); Beets; Carrots; Chrysanthemum (Garland); Chrysanthemum Leaves; Cucumber with peel; Endive; Epazote; Fennel (Bulb); Grape leaves; Hearts of palm; Kelp; Various Lettuce; Nopal; Shallots; Various Squash; Sweet potatoes leaves; Taro; Tomatoes (sun-dried); Wasabi root; Brussels sprouts; Broccoli (Chinese); Radishes; Zucchini; Mustard greens; Eggplant; Kale; Garlic; Mushrooms; Turnips; Collards; Pumpkin; Rutabaga; Cauliflower;

Breads, Grains, Cereals, Pasta

Cereal (corn flakes); Cereals: rice crisps, shredded wheat, whole-wheat; English muffins (whole-wheat); Other Cereals; Bagels; Breads: French/Sourdough, Italian; English muffins; Tortillas (corn); Spaghetti (whole-wheat); Amaranth; Buckwheat; Quinoa; Toasted bread; Various Rolls; Crackers (whole-wheat); Biscuits; Waffles; Bulgur; Triticale; Various Breads; Crackers (saltines); Rice (white); Spaghetti; Rice (wild); Spelt; Oatmeal (cereal); Whole-wheat; Durum wheat; Rye grain; Sorghum grain; Various Crackers; Pasta; Semolina; Wheat; Bread sticks; Couscous; Melba toast; Wheat bran; Rice (brown); Muffins (wheat bran);

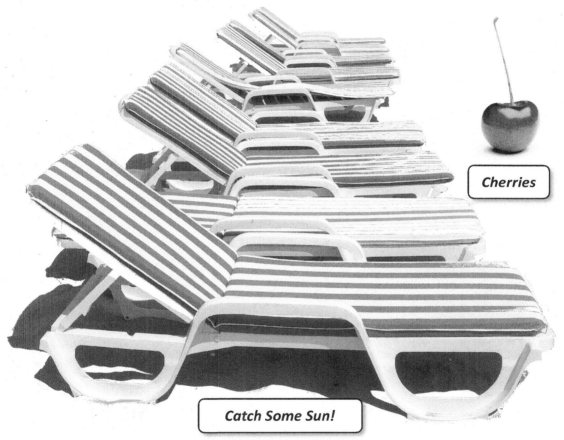

**Cherries**

**Catch Some Sun!**

Dairy Products, Fats & Oils

Fish oil (cod liver); Milk (1% fat); Milk (skim); Fat-free or low fat dairy products; Cheese (Cottage); Whey (sweet); Cream; Yogurt; Buttermilk; Milk: 2% fat, whole; Cheese (Ricotta); Sour cream;

Desserts, Snacks, Beverages

Water; Popcorn (air popped); Coffee (decaf; lowers gout risk among men); Pretzels; Potato chips; Popcorn (oil popped); Tortilla chips; Coffee; Pie crust;

Herbs & Spices, Fast Foods, Prepared Foods

Cornmeal (whole-grain); Tofu; Potato pancakes; French fries; Egg rolls (veg); Macaroni; Parsley; Taco shells; Hash brown potatoes; Corn salad; Croutons; Thyme (fresh); Onion rings; Pizza;

Alternative Therapies & Miscellaneous

Exposure to Sun (limit to ten minutes per day); **Fluids/Juices/Water**; Exercise;

Key Nutrients & Herbal Meds

Vitamin D; Celery seed; Starch/complex Carbohydrates;

<u>Do not</u> choose these for Gout & Vitamin D Deficiency

Top 5 items to avoid:

Excess Body Weight; Cured & Luncheon Meats; Chocolate; Beer & Brewer's Yeast; 2+ Alcoholic Drinks/Day; Fasting;

Avoid or consume much less of the following (within a food group, most harmful items are listed first):

Meat, Fish & Poultry

Cured Meats; Beef jerky sticks; Salami; Bologna; Corned beef; Frankfurters; Luncheon meats; Pastrami; Pepperoni; Pork liver cheese; Sausages; Bacon; Pork breakfast strips; Pork cured/ham; Chorizo; Caviar; Scallops; Organ Meats; Salmon (smoked, Lox); Beef (ground); Beef chuck/brisket; Chicken & Turkey skin; Lamb ribs; Goose; Lamb leg; Pork ribs; Anchovy; Fish roe; Pheasant; Quail; Veal loin; Veal shoulder; Pheasant breast; Quail breast; Pork; Beef; Chicken dark meat; Shrimp; Tuna (canned); Pork skins; Bison/buffalo meat; Chicken; Duck (no skin); Rabbit meat; Venison; Lamb; Chicken breast (no skin); Cod; Haddock; Lobster; Mussels; Squid (Calamari); Chicken wings; Game Meat; Squab (pigeon); Turkey dark meat; Northern pike; Tuna (yellowfin); Walleye; Goat meat; Guinea hen; Turkey breast; Herring; Oysters; Sardines; Veal shank; Frog legs; Snail; Sablefish; Perch; Clams; Croaker; Crayfish; Abalone; Conch; Various Crab; Cuttlefish; Lobster (spiny); Octopus; Whelk; Various Bass; Bluefish; Burbot; Butterfish; Cisco; Cusk; Dolphinfish (Mahi-Mahi); Drum; Grouper; Ling; Lingcod; Mackerel (king); Milkfish; Monkfish; Orange roughy; Pollock; Pout; Pumpkinseed sunfish; Scup; Seatrout; Shark; Sheepshead; Smelt; Spot; Sucker; Tilefish; Turbot; Wolffish; Yellowtail; Flatfish (flounder & sole); Halibut; Tuna (blue fin); Surimi; Mullet; Whiting;

Instead <u>choose</u>: Cisco (smoked); White fish (smoked); Rockfish; Tilapia; Mackerel;

Eggs, Beans, Nuts and Seeds

Soybeans (dried); Peas (split); Cashew nuts; Beans (lima); Lentils; Coconut meat (dried); Soybeans (green); Alfalfa sprouts; Lupin; Pigeon peas; Coconut meat (raw); Various Beans; Black-eyed peas; Seeds (sunflower); Pili nuts; Chickpeas; Coconut milk; Peas (green); Peanuts;

Instead <u>choose</u>: Almonds; Hazelnuts or Filberts; Pecans; Egg (duck); Egg (hard-boiled); Egg (raw); Various Seeds; Acorns; Beechnuts; Egg substitute; Egg white; Pine nuts; Pistachio nuts; Walnuts; Peas (sugar/snap); Beans: yardlong, fava, hyacinth, navy, winged; Breadfruit seeds; Butternuts; Chestnuts; Ginkgo nuts; Hickory nuts; Macadamia nuts; Brazil nuts;

Fruits & Juices

Avoid sugared fruit juices or from concentrate;

Instead <u>choose</u>: Passion fruit; Apricots; Apricots (dried); Banana (dried);

Vegetables

Asparagus;

Instead *choose*: **Artichoke; Leeks; Green beans; Spinach;**

Breads, Grains, Cereals, Pasta

Danish pastry; Sweet rolls; Donuts; Muffins (blueberry); Corn; Noodles (egg); Muffins (oat bran); Barley;

Instead *choose*: **Cereal (granola); Oats Millet; Muffins (corn); Other Noodles; Oat bran; Rice bran; Rice cakes (Brown rice); Spaghetti (spinach); Wheat germ; Granola bars; Croissant;**

Dairy Products, Fats & Oils

Milk (chocolate); Hydrogenated vegetable oil; Vegetable shortening; Margarine; Oils: Babassu, coconut, Ucuhuba Butter, Cocoa Butter, Cupu Assu; Fat (beef/lamb/pork); Oils: palm, Shea nut; Fat (duck); Fish oil (menhaden); Lard; Cheese (American);

Instead *choose*: **Other Cheese; Cheese spread; Cream (whipped); Other Fish Oil; Other Oils; Margarine-like spreads; Non-dairy creamers; Butter;**

Desserts, Snacks, Beverages

Coffee liqueur; Red Bull (drink); Hot chocolate; Ice cream (chocolate); Cookies (chocolate chip); Chocolate (dark); Cake (chocolate); Chocolate mousse; Soft (carbonated) drinks; Chocolate (sweet); Beer; Applesauce; Cream puffs/Éclair; Crème de menthe; Molasses; Puff pastry; Carob (candy); Dessert toppings; Candies (peanut bar); Brownies; Ginger ale; After-dinner mints; Cheesecake; Chewing gum; Peanut butter; Piña colada; 80+ proof distilled alc. bev.; Fruit punch; Lemonade; Whiskey; Candies; Coffeecake; Halvah (candy); Various Pies; Eggnog; Frostings; Jams & Preserves; Jellies; Marshmallows; Pudding; Sherbet; Cookies; Tonic water; Cakes; Sports drinks; Fruit leather/rolls; Ice cream (vanilla); Ice cream cones; Frozen yogurt; Honey; Milk shakes; Pancakes; Taro chips; Tea (plain);

Instead *choose*: **Wine (red); Wine (white); Potato sticks; Tea (herbal); Malted drinks (nonalcoholic); Tea (green);**

Herbs & Spices, Fast Foods, Prepared Foods

Hot dog; Syrup (chocolate); Foie gras or liver pate; Teriyaki sauce; Beef broth & stock; Chicken broth & stock; Barbecue sauce; Tempeh; Tofu (fried); Fish stock; Gravies (canned); Sugars; Syrups; Miso; Soy sauce; Salad dressings; Chicken Nuggets; Pickle (sweet); Tahini; Soups: beef barley, chicken noodle, veg/beef; Cocoa; Ketchup; Soup (clam chowder); Sauce (Hoisin); Sausage (meatless);

Instead *choose*: **Hush puppies; Kimchi; Potato salad; Nachos; Cole slaw; Dill weed; Sage; Sauerkraut; Breaded shrimp; Balsamic vinegar; Herbs & Spices; Capers; Horseradish; Mayonnaise; Mustard; Pickle (cucumber); Sauces; Sugar (maple); Tomato paste; Vinegar; Cheeseburger; Hamburger; Falafel; French toast;**

Alternative Therapies & Miscellaneous

Excess body weight (avoid low carb diets); **2+ alcoholic drinks/day**; **Fasting (for a specific period, don't skip meals)**; Aspirin; Corn syrup; Deep-fried foods; Smoked fish/foods; High dosages of Niacin; Prescription drugs (diuretics such as thiazide);

Key Nutrients & Herbal Meds

Brewer's Yeast; Alcohol; Purine; Sugar (fructose); Sugar (refined); Caffeine;

References

All the material and suggestions presented in this book are based on the content available at PersonalRemedies.com. The primary sources used by that web site and therefore this book are US government sources. For complete and detailed information about all the references please visit PersonalRemedies.com.

The suggestions provided are derived from, confirmed by, or based on a long list of references, some of which are listed below. This list does not represent a complete or comprehensive list of all references used. Some references such as the US Government sources are relied upon more than others.

- USDA (US Department of Agriculture). Most of the nutrient data used by Personal Remedies and thus this book are based on USDA publications.
- National Institute of Health (NIH) of the United States. Most of the health information and the relationship between various nutrients and various health conditions are based on NIH and its various publications and agencies.
- NIH - Office of Dietary Supplements Web site.
- MedlinePlus Health Information - a service of National Library of Medicine and NIH.
- NIH - National Institute of Arthritis and Musculoskeletal and Skin Disease
- NIH - National Center for Complementary and Alternative Medicine (NCCAM)
- Dept. of Health and Human Services. Centers for Disease Control and Prevention.
- National Cancer Institute.
- National Diabetes Information Clearinghouse (NDIC). A Service of National Institute of Diabetes and Digestive and Kidney Diseases (NIDDK) and NIH.
- National Kidney and Urologic Diseases Information Clearinghouse (NKUDIC). A service of the National Institute of Diabetes and Digestive and Kidney Diseases (NIDDK), National Institutes of Health (NIH)
- PRAL (Potential Renal Acid Load) formula applied to USDA nutrient database data
- The President's Council on Physical Fitness and Sports.
- US Dept. of Health and Human Services; US Environmental Protection Agency
- Dash Eating Plan; Your Guide to Lowering Blood Pressure with Dash; US Dept. of Health and Human Services; NIH; National Heart, Lung and Blood Institute
- National Heart, Lung and Blood Institute
- Office on Women's Health; US Dept. of Health and Human Services

Secondary sources used by that site include:

- American Heart Association (www.heart.org)
- Institute of Medicine - Food and Nutrition Board - Dietary Reference Intakes. (www.iom.edu)
- *Dietary Reference Intakes - The essential Guide to Nutrient Requirements* (Institute of Medicine of the National Academies. The National Academies Press. 2006)

- *The PDR Family Guide to Natural Medicines & Healing Therapies* (Ballantine Books; New York. First Edition; May 2000)
- *The PDR Family Guide to Nutritional Supplements* (Ballantine Books; New York; 2001)
- MayoClinic.com. Reliable information for a healthier life from Mayo Clinic (www.mayoclinic.com)
- Harvard School of Public Health (www.hsph.harvard.edu)
- American Cancer Society (www.cancer.org)
- American Academy of Physical Medicine and Rehabilitation (www.aapmr.org)
- American Diabetic Association (www.diabetes.org)
- American Dietetic Association (www.eatright.org)
- Multiple Sclerosis Society (www.nationalmssociety.org)
- *The American Pharmaceutical Association Practical Guide to Natural Medicines*. (Andrea Pierce; Morrow; 1999)
- Living Well With HIV/AIDS - A manual on nutritional care and support for people living with HIV/AIDS. Food and Agriculture Organization of the United Nations
- Stanford Hospital & Clinics. Low FODMAP diet handout
- The University of Arizona Campus Health Service. The Low FODMAPs Diet.
- Crohn's & Colitis Foundation of America
- www.herpes.com
- Australian Institute of Sports (www.ais.org.au)
- www.healthandage.com (Sponsored by Boomerang Pharmaceutical Communications)
- www.essense-of-life.com
- Gout (Prof. R. Grahame, Dr. A. Simonds and Dr. E. Carrey); and www.acumedico.com
- Environmental Working Group (www.EWG.org)
- International Foundation for Functional Gastrointestinal Disorders, Inc. (IFFGD), and Monash University, creators of low FODMAP diet for IBS
- Sjögren's Syndrome Foundation (www.sjogrens.org)
- The Dark Side of Wheat (by Sayer Ji; www.GreenMedInfo.com)
- www.GreenMedInfo.com
- High pH therapy research by A.K. Brewer, and Nobel prize winner Otto Warburg (BREWER, A. K. The high pH therapy for cancer tests on mice and humans)
- Linus Pauling Institute Micronutrient Research for Optimum Health
- *Eat Well, Live Well with Spinal Cord Injury* (Joanne Smith and Kylie James; 2013)
- The Oxalate Content of Food By Helen O'Connor, MS, RD
- Oxalate Content of Foods. The Children's Medical Center (Dayton's Children)
- The Oxalosis & Hyperoxaluria Foundation
- New York University (NYU) Langone Medical Center

For Additional Information

For personal food list suggestions for

- other health conditions,
- other combinations of health conditions,
- a greater list of food choices,

and for more detailed nutrition information, you may wish to look at other books in our *Choose This not That* series listed at the end of the book or visit PersonalRemedies.com.

Acknowledgements

We would like to thank the following individuals for their support, encouragement, advice and contributions to the production of this book and contents of the Personal Remedies knowledgebase which is presented in this book: Ester Awnetwant-Esperon, MS, RD, LD; Karen Chiacu-Recco; Kate Fletcher-King; Amanda King; Avirat Kulkarni; Barbara Langathianos; Andrew Lenhardt, MD; Sih Han Lim; Mark Lu, MD; Steve Manson; Art McCray; Dick Neville; Christian Seeber; Nancy Elizabeth Shaw; Diana Silk; Scott Silk; George Sprenkle; Shahin Tabatabaei, MD; Katya Tsaioun, PhD, LD; Foad Vafaei; Rolie Zagnoli; Mory Bahar.

Personal Remedies, LLC

and

Simple Software Publishing

Who is Personal Remedies?

Personal Remedies is the largest producer of health & nutrition apps, books and eBooks for chronic conditions, in the market. Its patented software & knowledgebase can enable organizations such as healthcare providers to deliver apps for personalized and actionable nutrition guidance to their patients suffering from one or multiple chronic conditions.

Who is Simple Software Publishing?

Simple Software Publishing is a small publisher established in 1996. Our passion is to explain complex matters in an easy to understand form. We also strive to minimize the use of paper for production and distribution of books.

Choose This not That Series of Books, eBooks and Apps

Choose This not That for:
- Breast Cancer
- Cancer Prevention
- Cervical Cancer
- Colon Cancer
- Esophageal Cancer
- Gout
- High Blood Pressure
- High Cholesterol
- High Triglycerides
- IBS (Irritable Bowel Syndrome)
- Lung Cancer
- Ovarian Cancer
- Pancreatic Cancer
- Prostate Cancer
- Rheumatoid Arthritis
- Stomach Cancer
- Ulcers
- Vitamin D Deficiency
- … please send us your suggestion!

In addition, we offer mobile apps for the following conditions: age-related macular degeneration (AMD), Alzheimer's disease, celiac disease, Crohn's disease, diabetes type-2, Dietary Guidelines for Americans, Dietary Guidelines for 50+, heart disease, herpes, kidney stones (oxalate), obesity, osteoarthritis, osteoporosis, and PCOS (Polycystic Ovary Syndrome).

How to Order

To order eBooks (on Kindle or Nook) or printed copies of this book, or to order any of our other books please visit Amazon.com, Barnes & Noble, or contact us by email at Publisher@PersonalRemedies.com or send your purchase order or payments to:

> Simple Software Publishing
> 5 Oregon Street
> Georgetown, MA 01833

To order a colorful Mobile App version of this book, please visit Apple App store, Google Play (Android), or Amazon App Store.

For suggestions for new books and comments please email us at Books@PersonalRemedies.com.

Progress Tracker

To monitor your progress, date and note your symptoms and relevant data such as uric acid level in your blood, weight, pain level, cholesterol level, blood pressure... We love to hear about your feedback and progress. Email us at Books@PersonalRemedies.com.

Notes